Lifting the Curse of Menstruation

A Feminist Appraisal of the
Influence of Menstruation
on Women's Lives

About the Editor

Sharon Golub is an associate professor of psychology at the College of New Rochelle and adjunct associate professor of psychiatry at New York Medical College. The menstrual cycle is her major area of research interest and she has written and presented papers on various aspects of menstruation. Dr. Golub is the editor of a recently published book entitled *Menarche*. She is currently President of the Society for Menstrual Cycle Research and is editor of *Women & Health*.

Lifting the Curse of Menstruation

A Feminist Appraisal of the Influence of Menstruation on Women's Lives

Sharon Golub, PhD, Editor

The Haworth Press
New York

Lifting the Curse of Menstruation: A Feminist Appraisal of the Influence of Menstruation on Women's Lives has also been published as *Women & Health,* Volume 8, Numbers 2/3, Summer/Fall 1983.

The Haworth Press, Inc., 28 East 22 Street, New York, NY 10010

Library of Congress Cataloging in Publication Data
Main entry under title:

Lifting the curse of menstruation

"Has also been published as Women & health, volume 8, number 2/3, summer/fall 1983"
—T.p. verso.
Includes bibliographical references.
1. Menopause. 2. Women—Physiology. I. Golub, Sharon. II. Women & health
[DNLM: 1. Menstruation. 2. Menstruation disorders—Psychology. 3. Psychophysiology.
WP 540 L722]
RG186.L47 1983   612'.662'01   83-12723
ISBN 0-86656-242-7

Lifting the Curse of Menstruation
A Feminist Appraisal of the Influence of Menstruation on Women's Lives

Women & Health
Volume 8, Numbers 2/3

CONTENTS

Contributors

Judith M. Abplanalp, PhD, Assistant Professor, Department of Psychiatry & Behavioral Sciences, The University of Texas, Medical Branch, 312 Administration Annex, Galveston, TX 77550.

Anthony W. Clare, MD, Professor, Department of Psychological Medicine, St. Bartholomew's Hospital Medical College, West Smithfield, London, England EC4.

Mona Eliasson, PhD, Director, Center for Research on Women, Uppsala University, Psychology Department, Box 227, S-75104, Uppsala, Sweden.

Mary Anna Friederich, MD, Clinical Associate Professor, Obstetrics, Gynecology, & Psychiatry, University of Rochester, School of Medicine and Dentistry, Rochester, NY 14623.

Sharon Golub, PhD, Associate Professor, Department of Psychology, College of New Rochelle, New Rochelle, NY 10801.

Randi Daimon Koeske, PhD, Statistician and Data Analysis Coordinator, Western Psychiatric Institute and Clinic, 4223 PCGC, Department of Psychiatry, University of Pittsburgh School of Medicine, 3811 O'Hara Street, Pittsburgh, PA 15213.

Nancy Reame, RN, PhD, Associate Professor of Parent-Child Nursing, School of Nursing, University of Michigan, 1335 Catherine Street, Ann Arbor, MI 48109.

Barbara Sommer, PhD, Lecturer, Department of Psychology, University of California, Davis, Davis, CA 95616.

Ann M. Voda, RN, PhD, Professor, College of Nursing, University of Utah, 25 S. Medical Drive, Salt Lake City, UT 84112.

Preface

Menstruation has a bad reputation in our culture. Despite the fact that the menstrual cycle is an integral part of every woman's life from about the age 13 until she is almost 50, menstruation is viewed as an illness or problem by large numbers of people. Witness the terms often used to describe menstruation: "the curse," "falling off the roof," "being unwell," "riding the rag," and "losing blood." Perhaps as a consequence of labeling menstruation as a disease, many women and men think of the menstruating woman as being disabled or suffering from some impairment of function. The purpose of this monograph is to present an up-to-date view of menstruation from a feminist perspective with some suggestions for future research.

Feminists are not necessarily immune to socio-cultural pressures or to the unquestioning use of the medical model. In the first paper, Randi Koeske makes an important point: not only has menstrual cycle research been tainted by sexism and assumptions of biological determinism, but even feminist researchers have to struggle to find a rational balance between a feminist perspective that acknowledges the obvious importance of physiological influences on women's bodies and the psychosocial factors that interact with them. Koeske goes on to discuss the many flaws in menstrual cycle research attributable to "taken for granted" assumptions—both conceptual and methodological—and she offers suggestions as to how menstrual cycle research can become more sophisticated, reliable, and valid.

Menarche, the onset of menstruation, is a dramatic event in most women's lives. It is a tangible, physical sign marking the transition to womanhood. Sharon Golub reviews the physiological aspects of menarche, including the effects of genetics, nutrition, exercise, and illness. Then, turning to the psychosocial, the ways in which the changes of puberty and menarche affect the adolescent girl's perception of herself and her life are discussed. Particular emphasis is given to the unique problems of the early maturing girl who seems to need more support than she is currently getting.

Many people are surprised to learn that the first commercially successful disposable sanitary napkin was not marketed until 1921. Before that women used menstrual rags, cloth diapers, or tampons made of paper, cotton, or wool. Nancy Reame takes a scientific look at menstrual health products. She describes the factors affecting normal variations in menstrual flow, health problems related to menstrual hygiene, and methods used to study tampon and napkin absorbancy in the laboratory. Implications for the development of minimum safety standards for menstrual hygiene products are also noted.

Since the menstrual cycle is such an obvious difference between the sexes, correlates of the cycle are regularly raised as evidence of women's inferiority and many people believe that women are victims of their repeatedly cycling biological systems. This leaves psychologists with the ever present challenge of trying to prove that menstruation does *not* impair women's ability to function. In her paper, Barbara Sommer reviews studies of the effects of the menstrual cycle on a wide range of behaviors: cognitive tasks, work, academic performance, and perceptual-motor tasks. Sommer finds that "the weight of the evidence argues against a menstrual cycle effect on behavior." It would be most unfortunate if, because of sexist assumptions, we were doomed to repeat these studies ad infinitum.

While arguing against the idea that menstruation is debilitating for most women, it is important for us to attend to the real problems that it may present. A majority of women do report unpleasant or uncomfortable symptoms associated with the premenstrual and menstrual phases of the cycle. Dysmenorrhea, or painful periods, are a fact of life for many women. Mary Anna Friederich addresses its causes, proper diagnosis, and current methods of treatment. Premenstrual symptoms also affect many women. When do these symptoms become "PMS" (premenstrual syndrome)? Judith Abplanalp attempts to define PMS and reviews research dealing with the efficacy of the different treatments that have been advocated for the alleviation of premenstrual symptoms. With PMS so much in the news in the last year or so, it is important for health professionals to be able to sort out the claims of cure objectively and scientifically.

It also seems important to differentiate between the experiences of normal women and women who are experiencing a neurotic or psychotic illness. Anthony Clare reviews the relationship between psychopathology and the menstrual cycle. He observes that a number of studies link a recurrence in psychotic illness with the premenstrual phase of the cycle, while only a few studies support a link between neurosis and premenstrual symptoms. Clare notes the flaws in many of these studies and also points out a possible double bind for women. If mentally ill women get "sicker" during the premenstrual phase of the cycle, aren't all women similarly affected? Or, on the other hand, are all women who complain of premenstrual symptoms neurotic? Care must be taken that women are not told once again, "It's all in your head." Clare concludes that psychopathology is but one factor that may contribute to dysmenorrhea or premenstrual tension.

Finally, Ann Voda and Mona Eliasson focus on menopause as a normal occurrence rather than as a deficiency disease. They discuss the questions often asked by menopausal women about the hot flash, vaginal and urinary problems, bone pain, depression or mood swings, and the use of estrogen replacement therapy. And these authors decry the dearth of woman-centered research data available about menopause today. One hopes that the papers in this monograph will stimulate such research.

On behalf of *Women & Health* I would like to thank the contributors for sharing their expertise. Knowledge about the menstrual cycle will help all women to better understand their bodies. Such knowledge will also help to dispel myths that discredit women's ability to function at "that time of the month," and will enable those involved in the health care of women to provide better informed, higher quality care.

Sharon Golub, PhD
Editor

Lifting the Curse of Menstruation

A Feminist Appraisal of the Influence of Menstruation on Women's Lives

Lifting the Curse of Menstruation: Toward a Feminist Perspective on the Menstrual Cycle

Randi Daimon Koeske, PhD

ABSTRACT. Lifting the curse of menstruation is examined as a process of freeing the imagination rather than rejecting the importance of biology. The defining features of the feminist and biomedical perspectives are discussed and an overview is offered of unexamined assumptions about women, the cycle, and the conduct of research which operate within modern scientific medicine. The real alternative to these unexamined assumptions is seen as the development of a revolutionary system of classification in which even the smallest unit of analysis is a multidimensional process. Suggestions are offered about the proper role of the feminist perspective in helping to free our imaginations and move us toward such an alternative paradigm.

Many researchers and practitioners committed to feminism have suggested that biases (i.e., unexamined assumptions) such as sexism and biological determinism characterize the medical and psychiatric literature on the menstrual cycle.* It would be comforting if we

---

*Although the suggestions and viewpoints in this paper are the author's, they owe much to both the ground-breaking work sponsored by the Society for Menstrual Cycle Research and the recently completed document, *Guidelines for Nonsexist Research* (McHugh, Koeske, Frieze et al., 1981), endorsed by Division 35 (Psychology of Women) of the American Psychological Association.

The Society for Menstrual Cycle Research was founded in 1980 by its first President, Alice Dan, of the University of Illinois, Circle Campus. The current President of the Society is Sharon Golub of The College of New Rochelle, New Rochelle, New York.

The *Guidelines for Nonsexist Research* were the result of two years of effort by a national Task Force of psychologists appointed by Division 35. The final document was endorsed by the Division in December of 1981. Copies of the *Guidelines* may be obtained by contacting the authors, c/o Department of Psychology, University of Pittsburgh, Pittsburgh, PA 15260.

1

could treat these unexamined assumptions as mere oversights, and encouraging if we could believe that biomedical researchers were eager to correct the "errors" pointed out to them by feminist critics.

Unfortunately, no such self-congratulations appear warranted. Instead, menstrual cycle researchers and practitioners committed to feminism find themselves grappling with their *own* tacit acceptance of the biomedical world view, and many harbor uncertainties about how to reconcile their commitment to the importance of psychosocial factors with the apparently overwhelming evidence of biological influence in women's lives.

It is my belief that, in order to develop a more humane and nonsexist system of health care for women, researchers and practitioners alike must train themselves to systematically recognize and reevaluate the basic assumptions of the biomedical world view. Acknowledgement of biological influence in women's lives is not, per se, inconsistent with feminism. It is biomedicine's tacit assumptions about the meaning and elemental nature of biological factors which must be challenged. The feminist perspective provides one important starting point for doing this.

What does the feminist perspective entail, then? In essence, it challenges the view that science is disinterested and looks for linkages between beliefs about women and the social and political forces affecting women's lives. It strives to understand the hidden justification for power differences contained in scientific medicine's assumptions about what is normal or proper for women, for the cycle, and for the conduct of research. The feminist perspective should *not* be viewed as an effort to explain biomedical "facts" by reference to cultural rather than biological forces. It should *not* be reduced to the reminder that social and psychological factors are important, or equated with the idea that biological influence is trivial. Instead, the feminist perspective should be recognized as a challenge to the very distinctions—mind/body, cognition/emotion, trait/context, doctor/patient, expert/layman—which provide the basis for modern medicine. Viewed in this way, the feminist perspective represents one pathway to a more complex and interactive (i.e., biosocial) approach to menstrual cycle study and health care.

To better realize its potential for transforming menstrual cycle research, the feminist perspective must become more fully developed, however. The first task of recognizing weaknesses within biomedicine has been achieved. Now it is time for feminist researchers and practitioners to turn their attention to developing a more sophisticated critique of scientific medicine—a critique which contains within it the seeds of an alternative paradigm. This paper offers an overview of lessons and issues for consideration necessary to move us closer to that goal.

UNDERSTANDING THE SCOPE OF THE MENSTRUAL CYCLE

Reaching a more feminist perspective on the menstrual cycle requires recognizing that the menstrual cycle's current biomedical meaning derives from concepts and conflicts central to the emergence of modern medicine, especially gynecology and psychiatry. The menstrual cycle has been connected closely with the nineteenth century battle between scientific and experiential conceptions of the body, with efforts to interpret female behavior in light of women's larger social role, with the financial battles between modern medicine and its alternatives, and with the emergence of "expert knowledge" in such fields as public health, social work, education, psychology, medicine, and psychiatry (cf. Smith-Rosenberg & Rosenburg, 1973; Barker-Benfield, 1976; Wood; 1973; Ehrenreich & English, 1973a; 1973b; 1978; Walsh, 1977 for documentation of these points). Taken together, these converging trends have resulted in a dominance of "outsider" views of the menstrual cycle over "insider" views, and a preference for scientific expertise over experience as the arbiter of truth (cf. Dan, 1982; Koeske, 1982).

Awareness of this larger historical framework on the menstrual cycle alerts researchers to the limitations and hidden agenda of scientific study, to the normative and correctional foundations of the scientific perspective, and to the power differentials lurking behind willingness-to-treat that have pervaded scientific medicine. These features color the entire field of menstrual cycle study, including the biology of the cycle, and the cycle's link to such areas as emotions, brain function, social behavior, and health or illness. But they are probably clearest in research attempting to demonstrate some link between the menstrual cycle (or a cycle-relevant biological state) and behavior, where the probable causal significance of the menstrual cycle is implied or suggested. It is to this special brand of menstrual cycle research that we now turn.

Taken-for-Granted Assumptions in Menstrual Cycle Research

Scientific medicine's study of the linkages between the menstrual cycle and behavior frequently presupposes a background of taken-for-granted assumptions. These assumptions represent biases because they are not explicitly stated and are themselves rarely subjected to scientific scrutiny or empirical test. They express instead the accumulated common experience of membership in Western culture and modern biomedicine.

Two types of taken-for-granted assumptions, conceptual and methodological, may operate in scientific studies of the menstrual cycle. Following discussion of these two sets of assumptions, we will turn to an examination of how these assumptions are translated into actual studies of menstrual cycle-behavior linkage.

Taken-for-granted conceptual assumptions. Three separate but interrelated assumptions involving the meaning and causal significance of variables often underlie menstrual cycle research. They are:

1. *A focus on context-free factors inside the organism.* Biological and psychological factors are viewed primarily as forces operating inside the organism. Although factors temporally removed (e.g., genetic inheritance, early childhood experience) may be viewed as the ultimate causes of present biological and psychological states, factors which have a more immediate temporal impact on such states (e.g., body fat, nutrition, stress, lifestyle, current role relationships, recent life events) are often underplayed or ignored. The result is a tendency to speak about states (e.g., hormone levels) or traits (e.g., conflict over sex-role, congestive vs. spasmodic symptom pattern) so as to reify them rather than preserve their process-like qualities and contexts. The most commonly encountered explanatory models focus on such states and traits as the *causes* of behavior.

2. *A strong acceptance of the individual difference model.* The heavy reliance on individual differences to explain cycle-related phenomena permits toleration of wide variability between individuals and fosters a tendency to view individual differences as the result of different internal states or traits. Less attention is focused on a systematic examination of the

contextual influences (whether biological, psychological, situational, or sociocultural) which may systematically account for many of these individual differences. The individual difference model also tends to accentuate or oversimplify small overlapping differences, reifying them into distinct types and often casting them as unidimensional opposites (e.g., menopause vs. menstruation).

3. *Implicit normative assumptions.* A number of interrelated normative assumptions operate within research on the menstrual cycle, establishing "healthy" and "ill" poles of behavior and physiological state. Female behavior consistent with traditional gender roles is often treated as unquestionably "healthy." Changeableness, emotionality, and rhythmicity are either viewed as inherently unhealthy, or are evaluated according to norms concerning how regularly, in what form, or to what degree fluctuations must occur to be considered "normal."

These normative assumptions may derive from the association of so-called "healthy" states and traits with valued roles or functions (e.g., high hormone levels with fertility), or from an implicit comparison with the more valued male (e.g., female emotionality vs. male rationality). They are often oversimplified and unidimensional, frequently derive from assumed rather than empirically verified notions of what exists and what is functional, and often directly contradict women's own experiences.

Taken-for-granted methodological assumptions. Two interrelated methodological assumptions involving the meaning and proper conduct of science underlie most menstrual cycle research. They are:

1. *A positivistic emphasis on facts and description.* Following an outmoded logical positivism, many researchers within biomedicine view science as the accumulation of facts and consider descriptive research as quintessentially scientific. Absent from this view of science are the sophisticated insights of recent methodologists, philosophers, and historians of science (e.g., Giddens, 1976; Mitroff & Kilmann, 1978; Rychlak, 1977; Mahoney, 1976; Kuhn, 1962; Lakatos & Musgrave, 1970; Weimer, 1976) who have pointed to the constructionist role of the theory in science and have demonstrated linkages

between the concerns of science and the values of the larger
society (e.g., Sampson, 1977; 1981; Archibald, 1978; Rowan, 1974).

2. *A reductionistic, ahistorical, and atomistic approach to scientific problems.* Consistent with analytic reductionism, a majority of biomedical researchers prefer laboratory-based investigations which focus on increasingly smaller bits of the
full phenomenon by isolating it from its surrounding context.
A preference for variables and methods which are considered
"objective", i.e., value-neutral and relatively error-free,
characterizes this approach. Within this perspective, biological or biochemical variables are considered more basic—i.e.,
more reliable and valid (*and* more likely to be causes rather
than effects)—than psychological or social variables, despite
evidence of their sensitivity to situational influences, their
rhythmic variations, and their measurement reactivity. Cap-
turing brief snapshots of time, rather than allowing processes
to unfold in context, represents the most common sampling
strategy.

Translation of Taken-for-Granted Assumptions into Menstrual Research

Three broad issues involving the translation of taken-for-granted
conceptual and methodological assumptions into specific menstrual
cycle studies are discussed below. These are: the choice of variables
and samples for study; the design of the research; and the labeling,
interpretation, and explanation of results. It must be emphasized that
these three analytically separable phases of a research project are, in
practice, inextricably interrelated.

The choice of variables and samples for study. The hidden assumptions discussed above are perhaps most clearly illustrated in
the choice and operationalization of variables in the typical menstrual cycle study. Vagueness and imprecision in the delimitation of
concepts and the development of measures abound.

1. *Conceptual imprecision: what are the concepts?* Parlee (1973)
has been most persuasive in discussing the "premenstrual syndrome" as a concept ill-suited to scientific study because of its
vagueness and over-inclusiveness. As a descriptive classification,
the premenstrual syndrome (Frank, 1931; Greene & Dalton, 1953)
does not differentiate correlates of the premenstruum on the basis of

either frequency (e.g., over time or within subpopulations) or probable causal mechanism (e.g., concomitant hormone state, indirect physiological process, self-perception, or societal labeling). The boundaries of the premenstrual phase are themselves imprecise and may include the time up to two weeks before the onset of menstruation.

Similarly, the published research contains little discussion of the significance of the many procedures for determining cycle phase. A variety of phase definitions have been used, some of which count forward and some of which count backward from critical cycle events like ovulation or the onset of bleeding (Rogel, 1980). Since each of these events is continuous over time rather than discrete, some arbitrariness is inevitable. More importantly, perhaps, it is not clear what should be made of vastly different cycle phases or total cycle lengths: is the 2 days prior to onset of menses equivalent when the total cycle length is 25 vs. 40 days or when the post-ovulatory "half" of the cycle is 12 days vs. 18? The eagerness to decompose the cycle into phases and the strong acceptance of individual differences may have resulted in too much willingness to compare cycles that differ across time, across context, and across women without deciding in what ways they really are comparable.

Other definitional dilemmas have also been reported. Research on spasmodic vs. congestive dysmenorrhea has not been able to consistently demonstrate the theoretical separability of the two types (e.g., Webster, 1980). A number of questions have also been raised about the overemphasis on negative states, moods, and behaviors occurring during the premenstruum (Parlee, 1973; Koeske, 1976; 1980), the postpartum period (Parlee, 1979), menopause (Koeske, 1982; Kincaid-Ehlers, 1982; Stimpson, 1982), menarche (Brooks-Gunn & Ruble, 1980), and other uniquely female experiences (Schilling, 1978; Sherif, 1980). These phenomena, it has been suggested, should be conceptualized and measured neutrally or in a manner which includes both positive and negative experiences.

The concern in raising these definitional and operational imprecisions is both substantive and methodological. Wide variation in definitions and measurement procedures may render apparently comparable findings inconsistent. Even more importantly, the development of sound theoretical explanation cannot proceed until some agreement about what is to be explained can be achieved.

2. *Measurement and sampling difficulties: how are concepts and procedures linked?* Questions of measurement reliability and validi-

ty have been curiously ignored by many menstrual cycle researchers. The literature is replete with studies which fail to report the reliability of the measures employed, to include multiple measures of the same construct, or to develop methods of convergence when measures conflict. Despite the prevalence of physiological measures in menstrual cycle research, few researchers have offered a sophisticated discussion of how random error or irrevelant cyclical variation is to be removed from the data (cf. Smolensky, 1980; Halberg, Halberg, Halberg, & Halberg, 1980; Koeske, 1981; Schilling, 1981). Little concern has been raised about the proper units of analysis or the appropriate degree of data sensitivity necessary to permit testing of relevant hypotheses. Without some agreement on these issues, it becomes impossible to decide if the results of two studies conflict on substantive grounds or merely because of differences in the units of measurement employed.

The choice of research participants, too, has often left unanswered the question of how concepts and measures relate. Because much of the research has been conducted on patient populations, findings may exaggerate the extent to which menstrual cycle problems characterize the average woman. Recent research on college women and other normal samples which has not found the kind of pathology or extremity of response reported earlier seems to confirm this (Golub, 1980; Golub & Harrington, 1981). But it is not yet clear why the earlier and later samples' results differ. Sampling differences of this sort should alert us to the operation of unrecognized variables which may affect the degree or type of reported experiences, not cause us to prematurely dismiss conflicting results as due to "individual differences" or methodological errors.

Selection of research design. As a number of critics and reviewers (Parlee, 1973, 1981; Koeske, 1980; 1982) have pointed out, menstrual cycle research has been characterized by an overabundance of inferentially weak study designs, e.g., one-shot, cross-sectional and/or retrospective studies in which the relevance of the menstrual cycle as a topic of study is neither disguised nor varied. This research tradition seems to reflect three fundamental confusions about the conduct of research.

1. *A failure to distinguish descriptive from hypothesis-testing designs.* The most common type of study is one which observes some pattern of covariation between variables (e.g., hormone levels and moods) and then interprets the cause of the covariation in post-hoc fashion (e.g., falling hormone levels produce changes in brain

MAO which produce depressed mood). Not only does most such research fail to demonstrate that the explanation provided is appropriate, it also lacks credibility because of its failure to measure intervening variables postulated as important (e.g., brain MAO levels), control for possible confounding variables (e.g., situational stressors), test the hypothesis against plausible alternatives (e.g., hormones trigger perceivable body changes which influence mood through beliefs about mood and body change), or consider the fit of the hypothesis with the bulk of available studies (e.g., the studies showing no clear covariation of moods with cycle phases).

Since control groups are rarely or improperly included and the temporal sequencing of important variables remains unevaluated, most menstrual cycle research fails to rule out important methodological confounds such as external events occurring at the same time, noncomparability of comparison groups on variables besides those thought to be relevant, or measurement reactivity due to awareness of being measured (cf. Campbell & Stanley, 1963). Perhaps the most troublesome problem is the failure of most menstrual cycle research to include more than a limited range of possible causal variables, e.g., biological *or* psychosocial causal variables, but not both, in the same study.

2. *An incomplete understanding of "control" groups and "controlling for" irrelevant variables.* Control or comparison groups may work insidiously in menstrual cycle research when they *are* included. Often they compare responses in one cycle phase or in one group with another which is assumed to be normative. Thus, females are compared with males, premenstrual with intermenstrual women, menopausal with menstruating women, or oral contraceptive users with nonusers. More often than not, use of these comparison groups represents a misapplication of the ''control'' group concept because each such group involves a simultaneous variation of *many* factors, not just one.

Compared to a non-pill group, for example, pill users may be more sexually active, younger, healthier, more middle class, or non-Catholic. Their experience of the cycle is likely to differ because it is more predictable and often symptomatically less severe. Anxiety about pregnancy is bound to be less and the cycle may be much less easily disrupted by stress (unless the user forgets to take her pills). Depending on the hypothesis under investigation, these other variables may be crucial or relatively unimportant. It behooves the researcher to evaluate the appropriateness of commonly used comparison groups for the research hypothesis at hand, to consider what normative assumptions may lurk beneath possible "control" group choices, and to explore the simultaneous use of multiple control/comparison groups which represent several points along a single continuum.

Problems with control groups are equally prominent in treatment studies. Relatively few researchers employ double-blind or placebo controls, and when they do, there is some likelihood that participants' "real" experimental condition will become apparent (to observers or participants) before the study's conclusion (cf. Cullberg, 1972). Menstrual cycle research, like most scientific medical research, relies on a naive conception of the placebo (cf. Jospe, 1978; Brody, 1977). It needs to move toward a more sophisticated view of placebos and the client-therapist relationship in order to properly evaluate the role played in *all* treatments by side effects, the availability of a plausible "treatment theory," and treatment-induced changes in self-observation, behavioral regularity, or a sense of controllability.

3. *A lack of attention to measurement reactivity: changes in the meaning of measures.* Measurement reactivity is a problem of special concern for menstrual cycle researchers because of the frequent use of repeated measurements or structured recall instruments (e.g., the MDQ). But discussions of its importance are rare in the published literature. Relatively few researchers have trained respondents to self-measure appropriately before beginning data collection, or assessed changes in self-measurement over time by the use of multiple "measurement control" groups. Little has been written by menstrual cycle researchers about regression to the mean (spontaneous remission) among women with a high level of current complaints or among women seeking or receiving treatment. The effects of repeated blood or urine sampling on various physiological measures, and the likelihood of respondents guessing the research hypothesis when repeated measurements are taken have also remained largely unexplored. This lack of attention often appears to reflect the assumption that the meaning of measures is not problematic, at least as long as certain *types* of measures (e.g., hormonal assays vs. self-reports) are used.

Some movement toward a more sophisticated understanding of measurement reactivity has occurred in recent years. Considerable attention has been directed to the fallibility (Ruble & Brooks-Gunn, 1979) and reactivity (Parlee, 1974) of retrospective symptom recall, especially when the relevance of the menstrual cycle is known, for example. But only limited information is available about individual differences in symptom reporting (e.g., Ruble, Brooks, & Clark, 1980; Matthews, 1982) and even less is known about the attentional processes and labeling issues involved in perceiving cycle-related body changes (cf. Voda, 1982). Until more elaborate theories of symptom perception emerge, it is not clear how much of self-report data is measurement error and how much systematic or meaningful variation.

The use of labels, explanations, and interpretation. The variety of problems mentioned above often become painfully obvious when we examine the labels, explanations, and intepretations most commonly found in menstrual cycle research. Loaded terms expressing implicit normative assumptions abound: hormonal "deficits" or "excesses," sex-role "conflicts," "empty nests," post-partum "blues," and midcycle "peaks" all serve to communicate both what is expected and what is valued in each case.

As suggested above, vaguely or inclusively defined concepts, poorly specified causal mechanisms, and an overabundance of post-hoc one-factor models render the majority of menstrual cycle hypotheses untestable. Since the same measure may be differently labeled or the same concept differently operationalized by any two researchers, many of the findings represented in the published literature are noncumulative. A variety of different interpretive schools exist side by side, each subscribing to a particular set of beliefs and dismissing competing beliefs on methodological grounds—not necessarily because theirs are better researched but because theirs share a common framework of untested assumptions.

Researchers need to move beyond this tendency to offer plausible global explanations which fit a selected set of findings and to invest more time in recognizing and testing implicit assumptions, searching for specific disconfirmations of theory, and engaging in cross-disciplinary debate about concepts and procedures. To do this, they will need to overcome two major obstacles to interdisciplinary dialogue.

1. *The absence of a shared cross-disciplinary framework of concepts.* Particularly destructive to cross-disciplinary and cumulative research is the absence of an agreed-upon system for classifying and interrelating variables. One consequence is that researchers trained in competing subdisciplines often differ widely in their understanding of where variables are located, what other factors influence

or are influenced by them, and how far their range of influence extends.

For example, a number of researchers interested in perception (e.g., Koeske, 1980; Parlee, 1974; Ruble, 1977; Ruble & Brooks-Gunn, 1979) have provided evidence that reports of or beliefs about body changes over the course of the menstrual cycle should not be equated with actual body changes. Instead, they should be treated as occurring at another level of complexity, a level often influenced by shared sociocultural beliefs and affected by psychologically meaningful cues such as distinctiveness, evaluative connotation, or contextual salience. This implies that reports of body changes should be complexly evaluated in both treatment studies and studies attempting to explain behavior or experience in biological terms. An oversimplified view of symptom reports may lead investigators to erroneously claim a treatment is biologically efficacious when it produces changed symptom perception, or to disregard the importance of perceptual or contextual factors in explaining body changes measured by self-report.

2. *The reliance on imprecise and overly deterministic causal models.* Similar problems of miscommunication between disciplines occur when the range of a variable's influence goes unspecified. Some variables (e.g., genetic predisposition, early childhood experiences) are believed to exert long-lasting influence but this influence is channeled and made salient by more immediate situational factors. Other variables (e.g., perceptual cues, specific drug treatments) may be thought of as exerting quite specific or localized effects. Researchers need to be clearer about detailing the range of influence a variable is likely to have. Moreover, they need to specify whether a variable's effects are direct or mediated (i.e., require other conditions to be met before they can exert their effects).

Of course, biologically oriented researchers are not the only ones who have failed to make necessary conceptual distinctions, have been imprecise in specifying exact causal mechanisms, or have exaggerated the range of influence their preferred causal variables are thought to exert. Psychologically and socioculturally oriented researchers have made similar errors. They have exaggerated the determinative effect that socialization (especially early socialization) has on experience. They have emphasized the powerful distorting effects of socialization on experience (by suggesting, for example, that women are socially conditioned to view menstruation negatively), while somewhat underplaying the ecological validity (''grain of truth'') and diversity within subcultures which may also characterize socialized beliefs.

Similarly, cultural variability has too often been traced to the impact of differential socialization, even when biological factors represent equally valid candidates for its explanation. Often, the exact mechanisms by which socialization exerts its effects have gone unspecified and an impression has been left that biological factors *cannot* be determinative if cultural variability exists. Following the lead of many biologically oriented researchers, many socioculturally oriented researchers have too readily restricted the impact of culture to the psychosocial arena of attitudes, beliefs, perceptions, role performances and traits, failing to consider its impact on biologically meaningful variables such as diet, health practices, parity, longevity, or the availability of gene pools (cf. Koeske, 1982). These problems ultimately restrict the appeal and testability of sociocultural theories.

FEMINISM AND THE FUTURE
OF MENSTRUAL CYCLE RESEARCH

The foregoing discussion of weaknesses in current menstrual cycle research points to the need for a more self-aware, thorough, and hypothesis-testing approach to menstrual cycle study. Feminism can contribute to this kind of science in a variety of ways. It can offer critical analyses, emphasize "insider" perspectives, and continue its commitment to alternative methods, epistemologies, and philosophies of science. It can also encourage clients and practitioners to relate on a more equal basis, emphasize care as well as cure, and explore non-medical and self-help forms of intervention.

But feminists must be clear about their role. Their perspective is not a simple adjunct to biomedicine. Neither should it be a repudiation of the role of biological factors in women's experiences, or an exclusive focus on psychological and sociocultural factors as these have been traditionally defined. The *real* alternative to biomedicine is a system of health research and health care which finds a way to reintegrate the whole person from the jigsaw of parts created by modern scientific medicine. The strength of the feminist perspective is its recognition that the parts biomedicine currently recognizes *cannot* be reassembled into a whole. The challenge of the future is nothing less than a new way of conceptualizing the person, the cycle, and the conduct of research. We must put aside the false dichotomies formalized by biomedicine in the nineteenth century and develop a system of classification in which even the smallest unit of analysis is a multidimensional process. A vital first step toward this goal is the struggle to unlock the hold of biomedical categories from our own thinking.

REFERENCES

Archibald, W. P. *Social psychology as political economy.* Toronto: McGraw-Hill Ryerson, 1978.

Barker-Benfield, G. J. *The horrors of the half-known life: Male attitudes toward women and sexuality in nineteenth-century America.* New York: Harper and Row, 1976.

Brody, H. *Placebos and the philosophy of medicine.* Chicago: University of Chicago Press, 1977.

Brooks-Gunn, J. & Ruble, D. Menarche: The interaction of physiological, cultural, and social factors. In A. J. Dan, E. A. Graham, C. P. Beecher (Eds.), *The menstrual cycle.* New York: Springer, 1980.

Campbell, D. T. & Stanley, J. C. *Experimental and quasi-experimental designs for research.* Chicago: Rand McNally, 1962.

Cullberg, J. Mood changes and menstrual symptoms with different gestagen/estrogen combinations. A double blind comparison with a placebo. *Acta Psychiatrica Scandinavica,* 1972, *51,* (Whole Supplement 236).

Dan, A. J. The Interdisciplinary Society for Menstrual Cycle Research: Creating knowledge from our experience. In A. M. Voda, M. Dinnerstein, & S. R. O'Donnell (Eds.), *Changing perspectives on menopause.* Austen: University of Texas Press, 1982.

Ehrenreich, B. & English, D. *Witches, midwives, and nurses: A history of women healers.* Old Westbury, N. Y.: The Feminist Press, 1973a. (Glass Mountain Pamphlet No.1)

Enrenreich, B. & English, D. *Complaints and disorders: The sexual politics of sickness.* Old Westbury, N. Y.: The Feminist Press, 1973b. (Glass Mountain Pamphlet No. 2)

Ehrenreich, B. & English, D. *For her own good: 150 years of the experts' advice to women.* Garden City, N. Y.: Doubleday/Anchor Press, 1978.

Frank, R. T. The hormonal causes of premenstrual tension. *Archives of Neurology and Psychiatry,* 1931, *26,* 1053-1057.

Giddens, A. *New rules of sociological method.* New York: Basic Books, 1976.

Golub, S. Premenstrual changes in mood, personality, and cognitive function. In A. J. Dan, E. A. Graham, & C. P. Beecher (Eds.), *The menstrual cycle.* New York: Springer, 1980.

Golub, S. & Harrington, D. M. Premenstrual and menstrual mood changes in adolescent women. *Journal of Personality and Social Psychology,* 1981, *41,* 961-965.

Greene, R. & Dalton, K. The premenstrual syndrome. *British Medical Journal,* 1953, *1,* 1007-1014.

Halberg, E., Halberg, J., Halberg, F., & Halberg, F. Infradian rhythms in oral temperature before human menarche. In A. J. Dan, E. A. Graham, & C. P. Beecher (Eds.), *The menstrual cycle.* New York: Springer, 1980.

Jospe, M. *The placebo effect in healing.* Lexington, MA: Lexington Books, 1978.

Kincaid-Ehlers, E. Bad maps for an unknown region: Menopause from a literary perspective. In. A. M. Voda, M. Dinnerstein, & S. R. O'Donnell (Eds.), *Changing persepectives on menopause.* Austen: University of Texas Press, 1982.

Koeske, R. D. Physiological, social and situational factors in the premenstrual syndrome. Unpublished manuscript, 1976.

Koeske, R. D. Theoretical perspectives on menstrual cycle research: The relevance of attributional approaches for the perception and explanation of premenstrual emotionality. In A. J. Dan, E. A. Graham, C. P. Beecher (Eds.), *The menstrual cycle.* New York: Springer, 1980.

Koeske, R. D. Theoretical and conceptual complexities in the design and analysis of menstrual cycle research. In P. Komnenich, M. McSweeney, J. A. Noack, & N. Elder (Eds.), *The menstrual cycle.* New York: Springer, 1981.

Koeske, R. D. Toward a biosocial paradigm for menopause research: Lessons and contributions from the behavioral sciences. In A. M. Voda, M. Dinnerstein, & S. R. O'Donnell (Eds.), *Changing perspectives on menopause.* Austen: University of Texas Press, 1982.

Kuhn, T. S. *The structure of scientific revolutions.* Chicago: University of Chicago Press, 1962.

Lakatos, I. & Musgrave, A. (Eds.). *Criticism and the growth of knowledge.* Cambridge: Cambridge University Press, 1970.

Mahoney, M. J. *Scientist as subject.* Cambridge, MA: Ballinger, 1976.

Matthews, K. A. & Carra, J. Suppression of menstrual distress symptoms: A study of Type A behavior. *Personality and Social Psychology Bulletin,* 1982, *8,* 146-151.

Mitroff, I. I. & Kilmann, R. H. *Methodological approaches to social science.* San Francisco: Jossey-Bass, 1978.

Parlee, M. B. Gaps in behavioral research on the menstrual cycle. In P. Komnenich, M. McSweeney, J. A. Noack, & N. Elder (Eds.), *The menstrual cycle.* New York: Springer, 1981.

Parlee, M. B. The premenstrual syndrome. *Psychological Bulletin,* 1973, *80,* 454-465.

Parlee, M. B. Stereotypic beliefs about menstruation: A methodological note on the Moos Menstrual Distress Questionnaire and some new data. *Psychosomatic Medicine,* 1974, *36,* 229-240.

Parlee, M. B. Psychological aspects of menstruation, childbirth, and menopause. In J. A. Sherman & F. Denmark (Eds.), *Psychology of women: Future directions of research.* New York: Psychological Dimensions, 1979.

Rogel, M. J. Analysis of data from menstrual cycles of unknown or unequal length. In A. J. Dan, E. A. Graham, & C. P. Beecher (Eds.), *The menstrual cycle.* New York: Springer, 1980.

Rowan, J. Research as intervention. In N. Armistead (Ed.), *Reconstructing social psychology.* Baltimore: Penguin, 1974.

Ruble, D. N. Premenstrual symptoms: A reinterpretation. *Science,* 1977, *197,* 291-292.

Ruble, D. N. & Brooks-Gunn, J. Menstrual symptoms: A social cognition analysis. *Behavioral Medicine,* 1979, *2,* 171-194.

Ruble, D. N., Brooks-Gunn, J., & Clark, A. Research on menstrual-related psychological states: Alternative perspectives. In J. E. Parsons (Ed.), *The psychobiology of sex differences and sex roles.* Washington, DC: Hemisphere Publishing, 1980.

Rychlak, J. F. *The psychology of rigorous humanism.* New York: Wiley, 1977.

Sampson, E. E. Scientific paradigms and social values: Wanted—a scientific revolution. *Journal of Personality and Social Psychology,* 1978, *36,* 1332-1343.

Sampson, E. E. Cognitive psychology as ideology. *American Psychologist,* 1981, *36,* 730-743.

Schilling, K. D. Views of normality of uniquely female experience. Paper presented at the Association of Women in Psychology Conference, Pittsburgh, March, 1978.

Schilling, K. M. What is a *real* difference? Content or method in menstrual findings. In P. Komnenich, M. McSweeney, J. A. Noack, & N. Elder (Eds.), *The menstrual cycle.* New York: Springer, 1981.

Sherif, C. W. A social psychological perspective on the menstrual cycle. In J. E. Parsons (Ed.), *The psychobiology of sex differences and sex roles.* Washington, DC: Hemisphere Publishing, 1980.

Smith-Rosenberg, C. & Rosenberg, C. The female animal: Medical and biological views of woman and her role in nineteenth-century America. *Journal of American History,* 1973, *6,* 332-356.

Smolensky, M. H. Chronobiologic considerations in the investigation and interpretation of circamensual rhythms. In A. J. Dan, E. A. Graham, & C. P. Beecher (Eds.), *The menstrual cycle.* New York: Springer, 1980.

Stimpson, C. R. The fallacy of bodily reductionism. In A. M. Voda, M. Dinnerstein, & S. R. O'Donnell (Eds.), *Changing perspectives on menopause.* Austen: University of Texas Press, 1982.

Voda, A. M. Menopausal hot flash. In A. M. Voda, M. Dinnerstein, & S. R. O'Donnell (Eds.), *Changing perspectives on menopause.* Austen: University of Texas Press, 1982.

Walsh, M. R. *Doctors wanted. No women need apply.* New Haven, CN: Yale University Press, 1977.

Webster, S. K. Problems for diagnosis of spasmodic and congestive dysmenorrhea. In A. J. Dan, E. A. Graham, & C. P. Beecher (Eds.), *The menstrual cycle.* New York: Springer, 1980.

Weimer, W. B. *Psychology and the conceptual foundations of science.* Hillsdale, N. J.: Lawrence Erlbaum Associates, 1976.

Wood, A. D. "The fashionable diseases": Women's complaints and their treatment in nineteenth-century America. *Journal of Interdisciplinary History,* 1973, *4,* 25-52.

Menarche:
The Beginning of Menstrual Life

Sharon Golub, PhD

ABSTRACT. Menarche represents a developmental milestone in a woman's life. This paper reviews current knowledge about the physiological aspects of menarche and its place in the sequence of pubertal development. Hypotheses regarding the mechanisms that trigger menarche are presented, as is our current understanding of the influence of hormones, genetic factors, nutrition, exercise, and illness. Also discussed are the ways in which the changes of puberty and menarche affect the adolescent girl's psychosocial development, the unique problems of the early maturing girl, and the kind of preparation for menarche that is needed.

In "The Curse of an Aching Heart," playwright William Alfred captures the significance of menarche in a woman's life. One of the characters, a woman in her sixties, recalls being frightened and embarrassed when she got her first period. She awoke with stained bed clothes and sheets and didn't understand what was happening to her. Confused, she ran out of the house and after walking for awhile she happened upon a neighbor who recognized that she was upset and invited her in for a cup of tea. The neighbor explained menstruation to the girl and then, in honor of the occasion, the woman gave the girl a brooch. In the play, memory of this event was poignantly related to another woman more than forty years later.

Is this vignette a fluke, a bit of a sentimental whimsy? Probably not. Psychological research confirms the dramatist's intuition that menarche is an important developmental event. In a study of recollections of menarche, Golub and Catalano (1983) found that almost all of the 137 women studied, ranging in age from 18 to 45, remembered their first menstruation. And a majority could describe

The author would like to thank Dr. Rita Jackaway Freedman and Dr. Leon M. Golub for their helpful comments on an earlier draft of this paper and Ms. Vera Mezzaucella for her ever-cheerful support and skilled typing of the manuscript.

17

in detail where they were when it happened, what they were doing, and whom they told. How many events in our lives are so vividly recalled?

It is surprising, therefore, that menarche has received so little research attention until quite recently. Now scientists have begun to look at both the physical and psychological aspects of menarche and at the ways in which they are inextricably linked. It is acknowledged that the changes of puberty do not occur in a psychosocial vacuum. Body changes affect a person psychologically and socially, and the person's life experiences influence the biological processes as well. Nowhere is this seen more clearly than at menarche. For example, what is the relationship between exercise and the onset of menarche? Do menarcheal experiences affect the later development of menstrual distress? What determines whether menarche is a stressful time for girls? What does the menarcheal experience mean to the pubertal girl? How does it affect the way she sees herself? Is there a relationship between menarche and sexual activity? And how soon after menarche is a young woman fertile? Although there is a great deal that we still do not know, this paper will address these questions and will review the highlights of what is known about the physiological and psychosocial aspects of menarche.

PHYSIOLOGICAL ASPECTS OF MENARCHE

Sequence of Pubertal Development

Menarche is preceded by characteristic body changes that occur some time between the ages of 9 and 16. Breast development usually, but not always, occurs first. There is an increase in body hair and there is also a weight gain, growth spurt, and a change in body proportions with the hips becoming fuller. Sweat glands become more active and a body odor develops that is thought to be related to an increase in sex hormone secretions from the adrenal gland. The skin becomes oilier, sometimes giving rise to skin problems. And while these external changes are going on there are concomitant changes occurring within the body: the uterus and vagina are growing (Grumbach, Grave, & Mayer, 1974; Katchadourian, 1977).

As noted above, breast development is usually the first sign of puberty with breast buds beginning to form around the age of 11. Breast development is influenced by the secretion of estrogen, particularly estradiol from the ovary, and probably by the secretion of prolactin from the anterior pituitary gland as well (Warren, 1983). There is a slight enlargement of the areolar and elevation of the breast as a small mound. Soon after, pubic hair begins to develop, usually at about age 11½. Axillary hair generally appears about two years after the beginning of pubic hair development. On the average, menarche occurs between 12.8 and 13.2 years. (For photographs and a detailed description of the stages of breast and pubic hair growth during puberty see Tanner, 1978.)

Pubertal development may be fast or slow. Some girls pass rapidly through the stages of breast and pubic hair development while others move slowly. On the average, the total time for the overall process of physical transformation from child to adult is about four years (Tanner 1978). However, some girls may take only 1½ years to pass through all the stages while the slower developers may take as long as five years to do so. For those working or living with girls in this age group it is important to keep in mind that there can be great variation in the normal time of onset and completion of pubertal development. It is perfectly normal for a girl to begin to menstruate any time between the ages of 9 and 16 and age mates may be at very different stages of sexual maturation—one 12 year old can look like a woman, another very much like a child.

There is a close relationship between menarche and the pubertal spurt in height. Girls start to menstruate after the growth spurt has peaked, when the rate of increase in height (height velocity) is falling. The growth spurt is nearly over at the time of menarche, with girls on the average growing only about two more inches after the onset of menstruation. However, some girls do grow as much as four inches more (Tanner, 1978).

Menarche marks a mature stage of uterine development but not reproductive maturity. Early cycles are often irregular and between 55 and 82 percent of menstrual cycles during the first two postmenarcheal years are anovulatory. Regular menstruation may not occur for several years. However, it is important to remember that despite the apparent absence of regular monthly ovulation, any individual cycle may be ovulatory and is potentially fertile (Brennock, 1982) as indicated by the fact that there were 30,000 pregnancies among girls under the age of 15 in the United States between 1973 and 1978. These teenagers are at high risk for pregnancy complications such as low birthweight, high infant mortality, and pregnancy induced hypertension (Leppert, 1983), in addition to the stressful social and psychological consequences of having a baby at 13 or 14 years of age.

What Triggers Menarche?

There is some controversy about what triggers menarche. Currently there are two hypotheses which relate menarcheal age to physical growth: one focusing on skeletal growth and the other on the accumulation of fat. The skeletal growth hypothesis is based on the idea that the premenarcheal girl must reach an appropriate stage of skeletal development in order to reproduce and, therefore, the age at which she reaches this structural status (mature height and pelvic dimensions) is closely correlated with menarcheal age (Tanner, 1978). The importance of skeletal maturity is related to the need for a body, specifically a pelvis, that is adequate in size to bear a child. And there is some data to support the idea that pelvic dimensions—an average biiliac diameter of 26.2 cms.—are significantly correlated with menarcheal age (Ellison, 1982). Thus menarcheal age is closely related to skeletal development and bone age can be used as an appropriate measure of developmental age in predicting when menarche will occur (Tanner, 1978). This view attributes the decline in average age at menarche during the last century (referred to in the literature as the secular trend) to the acceleration of skeletal growth during this time, presumably related to better nutrition and health. In contrast, slow skeletal growth, resulting from poor nutrition or high altitude, leads to delay in the onset of menstruation.

An alternative hypothesis, proposed by Frisch (1980), suggests that the onset of menstruation is contingent upon the accumulation of fat and that a critical minimum weight for height is necessary to trigger and maintain ovulation and menstruation. Frisch's explanation of the secular trend in menarcheal age is that girls reach 101 to 103 pounds, the average weight at menarche, sooner now, and therefore menstruation begins earlier. She points out that a late menarche is associated with slower increases in body weight such as that seen in cases of malnutrition, or among twins, because they grow more slowly. Frisch notes that the greatest change during the adolescent growth spurt up to the time of menarche is a 120 percent increase in body fat. At menarche, girls' bodies average about 24 percent fat, not much different from the 28 percent fat found in the average 18 year old woman. In contrast, boys at about 18 years of age are much leaner with 14 percent fat. Frisch theorizes that reproduction requires energy and the function of the stored fat is to provide readily accessible energy should it be needed for pregnancy and lactation.

In a recent study entitled, "Skeletal Growth, Fatness, and Menarcheal Age," Ellison (1982) compared the two hypotheses using factor analysis of longitudinal growth data on 67 middle-class white girls born in 1928 and 1919 and drawn from the Berkeley Guidance Study. Ellison found that height velocity prior to menarche was the strongest independent correlate of menarcheal age, accounting for over 50 percent of the variance. The weight factor made the second largest contribution, accounting for 18 percent of the variance in menarcheal age. Thus while there seems to be a strong relationship between adolescent weight and menarcheal age, its effect is apparently less than that of the skeletal development. Ellison makes the point that since skeletal growth tends to cease soon after menarche, natural selection would delay menarche until the pelvis could handle reproduction.

Hormones

Although incompletely understood, significant hormonal changes occur at puberty. The gonadal, adrenal, and hypothalamic-hypophyseal hormones are of major importance. It is the interrelationship of these hormones that later control the female reproductive cycle. However, endocrinologists now believe that the hormonal changes associated with sexual maturation actually begin at the time of conception. By the third trimester of pregnancy, the negative feedback system is established. (See Figure 1.) During infancy the hypothalamic gonadotropin regulating mechanism is "set" at a low level and remains there until around the time of puberty when there is an increase in the secretion of follicle stimulating hormone (FSH) and luteinizing hormone (LH) and a decrease in hypothalamic sensitivity. Put another way, the hypothalamic set point increases inducing a subsequent increase in the secretion of FSH, LH, and gonadal hormones (Petersen & Taylor, 1980).

The adolescent growth spurt is a result of the joint action of androgens and growth hormone (Tanner, 1978). A progressive increase in plasma dehydroepiandosterone and dehydroepiandosterone sulfate, which are weak androgens, begins at about eight years of age and continues through ages 13 to 15. These hormones, thought to originate from the adrenal gland, are the earliest hormonal changes to take place at puberty (Warren, 1983). They and

MENSTRUAL CYCLE HORMONE FEEDBACK SYSTEM

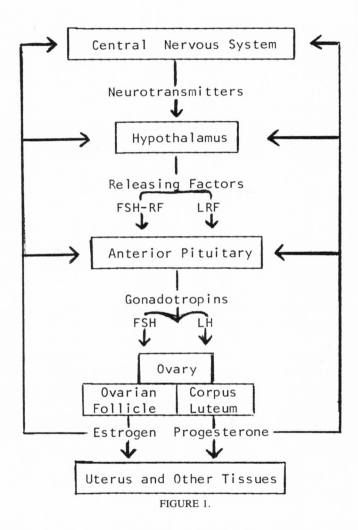

FIGURE 1.

the more potent androgens—testosterone and dihydrotestoster-
one—increase significantly as pubertal development progresses
(Dupon & Bingel, 1980). Increased secretion of gonadotropins from
the pituitary (FSH and LH) and sex steroids from the gonads follow
(Warren, 1983).

The main female sex hormone secreted by the ovaries is estradiol which is present in relatively small amounts in the blood until about age eight or nine when it begins to rise. This increase in blood levels of estradiol causes growth of the breasts, uterus, vagina, and parts of the pelvis. When menstruation begins, estradiol levels fluctuate with the various phases of the cycle and are controlled by pituitary FSH (Tanner, 1978).

The two pituitary gonadotropins, follicle stimulating hormone (FSH) and luteinizing hormone (LH), are both secreted in small amounts during childhood and increase at puberty. The pubertal rise is first seen as pulses of LH that are released during sleep. This sleep-associated rise in LH is not seen in either the prepubertal child or the adult (Warren, 1983). Gradually LH is released during the daytime too.

Menstruation, as well as earlier pubertal development, is thought to begin with a signal to the hypothalamus from the central nervous system. As noted above, a hypothalamic feedback system does exist before puberty, but the hypothalamus is responsive to low levels of LH in the prepubertal girl. Then around the time of menarche, a gradual change occurs making the hypothalamus less sensitive. Higher levels of estrogen are needed. The hypothalamus then secretes more FSH-releasing hormone. This neurohormone stimulates the pituitary glad to release FSH, which, in turn, triggers the growth of the ovarian follicle. As the follicles grow they secrete estrogen which causes growth of the cells lining the uterus (the endometrium). Increasing levels of estrogen in the blood also signal the pituitary to reduce FSH and secrete LH. LH triggers the release of the ovum from the follicle which then evolves into the corpus luteum and secretes progesterone and a little estrogen. If the ovum is not fertilized, the pituitary stops production of LH, levels of both estrogen and progesterone drop, menstruation begins, and the cycle starts again. (See Figure 1.)

Other Factors Affecting Pubertal Development

Genetics. Genetic factors play an important role in determining rate of growth, pubertal development, and age at menarche. Studies of monozygotic twin sisters growing up together indicate that they reach menarche about two months apart, with the first born twin— for some unknown reason—more likely to menstruate first (Shields, 1962). Dizygotic twins differ by about 12 months (Tanner, 1978).

Mother-daughter and sister-sister correlations have also been reported to be significant (Chern, Gatewood, & Anderson, 1980). Kantero and Widholm (1971) found other menstrual similarities between mothers and daughters: significant correlations were found between mothers' and daughters' length of cycle, duration of menstrual flow, and symptoms of dysmenorrhea and premenstrual tension. It is thought that both mother and father exert an equal influence on rate of growth and maturation. Thus a late-maturing girl is as likely to have a late-maturing father as a later-maturing mother (Tanner, 1978).

Nutrition. There is a well documented link between nutrition and fertility. Famine amenorrhea was reported in both world wars (Menkin, Watkins, & Trussell, Note 1). Young women who are undernourished because of excessive dieting or those with anorexia nervosa often do not have menstrual periods. And it is well known that malnutrition retards growth and will delay menarche (Tanner, 1978). The fall in age at menarche that has occurred between 1830 and 1960 coincides with the increased availability of protein in the diet of developed countries during this time. In some countries, where nutrition has remained inadequate, age of menarche is comparatively high. For example, in contrast with the average age of menarche in the United States, which is now 12.8 years, in Bangladesh it is just under 16, and among certain New Guinea tribes, it is about 18 (Menkin, Watkins, & Trussell, Note 1). A recent study by Goodman, Grove, and Gilbert (1983) in which no differences in age at menarche were found among Caucasian, Japanese, and Chinese women living in Hawaii, suggests that nutrition and environmental factors are responsible for population differences. Tanner (1978) has noted that children in urban, as opposed to rural, areas are more likely to have more rapid growth and an earlier menarche that is probably attributable to better nutrition, health, and sanitation.

Exercise. Exercise also affects menstruation. Women who experience high energy outputs, such as ballet dancers and athletes who train intensively, have a later age at menarche and a high incidence of amenorrhea. This is particularly true when intensive training begins at an early premenarcheal age (Frisch, 1980; Frisch et al., 1981; Frisch, 1983). It is not known whether an altered lean-fat ratio is responsible for the delay in menarche in young athletes, as proposed by Frisch, or if the delay occurs through the direct effects of exercise on hormonal secretion and metabolism (Rebar &

Cumming, 1981). Some investigators have questioned whether delays in the age of menarche in athletes occur at all (Malina, 1982). Others have expressed concern about the short-term and long-term effects of exercise on reproductive function (Rebar & Cumming, 1981). Also at this time it is not known whether it is disadvantageous to have a later menarche rather than an early one. However, the consensus seems to be that exercise-related alterations in reproductive function are not serious and are readily reversible.

Climatic and seasonal effects. Climate has no more than a very minor effect on age at menarche. In fact, contrary to earlier beliefs, people who live in tropical countries are somewhat more likely to have a *late* menarche. This is thought to be related to nutrition rather than a climate because children in the higher socioeconomic groups in these countries experience menarche at about the same time as children living in temperate zones.

Season of the year does influence growth velocity, with peak growth seen between March and July, and girls are most likely to have their first menstruation in the late fall or early winter (Science News, 1980; Tanner, 1978).

Acute and chronic illness. There are some conditions where menstruation will not occur. For example, a child with Turner's Syndrome, a chromosomal anomaly in which the second X chromosome is absent, will not menstruate because she lacks ovaries. Ehrhardt and Meyer-Bahlberg (1975) advise that sex hormone administration is crucial in order for these girls to attain psychosocial and psychosexual maturity. Administration of estrogen will cause the breasts to grow and an artificial menstrual cycle may be produced by giving estrogen for three weeks followed by a week without treatment. This is important because these girls want to look, develop, and be treated like normal female adolescents.

Other illnesses can delay menarche, probably because of their effects on nutrition. This is most likely to be true in cases of uremia, regional enteritis, ulcerative colitis, congenital heart disease, cystic fibrosis, and diabetes mellitus. The timing of the onset of the illness as well as the illness per se seem to be important. For example, if diabetes develops during the initial pubertal period, menarche is delayed, whereas if it develops later, menarche may be unaffected (Warren, 1983).

Conversely, some conditions will advance the age of menarche. These include hypothyroidism, central nervous system tumors, encephalitis, head trauma, and some virilizing disorders. Inactive, retarded, or bedridden children also reach menarche at an earlier age than their more active counterparts. And blind children have a younger age at menarche that may be related in part to their limited activity (Warren, 1983).

Thus menarche occurs after a series of changes in hormone secretion and somatic growth. These processes are in turn influenced by genetic and environmental factors such as nutrition, exercise, and illness which may accelerate or retard the onset of menstruation. We now turn to the psychosocial aspects of menarche and its meaning to the adolescent girl and those around her.

PSYCHOSOCIAL ASPECTS OF MENARCHE

Effects of Menarche on the Early Adolescent Girl

Much of the early writing about the psychology of menarche presented it as a traumatic experience. For example, early psychoanalytic theory postulated a marked increase in sex drive at puberty and an inevitable period of anxiety, worry about impulse control, and increased lability as "a relatively strong id confronts a relatively weak ego" (A. Freud, 1946). Benedek (1959) believed that menarche might evoke fears associated with the anticipation of pain during intercourse and childbirth. Current psychoanalytic views are much more positive. Notman (1983) and others suggest that meeting the developmental tasks of adolescence need not be as tumultuous as was previously believed. True, the early adolescent needs to modify her attachment to her parents and develop the capacity to form relationships with peers; and eventually she must establish her identity as a woman and develop the capacity for intimacy with another person. However, this need not happen overnight and the process should not cause turmoil or disintegration.

Menarche can have an organizing effect for the adolescent girl, helping her to clarify her perception of her own genitals, particularly confirming the existence of the vagina and correcting the confusion she may have had about the female genitalia. Kestenberg (1965) suggests that menarche may serve as a reference point around which girls can organize their pubertal experiences; it is a landmark for feminine identification. This is in keeping with the greater awareness of sexual differentiation between males and

females among postmenarcheal girls demonstrated by Koff, Rierdan, and Silverstone (1978).

Knowledge, Attitudes, and Expectations
in Anticipation of Menarche

What do the girls themselves say? Whisnant and Zegans (1975)
interviewed 35 white middle class pre- and postmenarcheal girls at a
summer camp. The girls had learned about menstruation from
friends, commercial booklets, school, and their parents—especially
their mothers. They perceived themselves as being knowledgeable
about menstruation and used the appropriate terms. However, when
questioned further the interviewer found that they really did not
have a good conception of what the internal organs were like or how
they functioned and they were even more inept at describing the external genitalia. Thus, despite their access to information about
menstruation, they had not assimilated it particularly well. The girls
were most concerned about what to do when they got their periods
and many had mentally rehearsed what they would do in a variety of
situations.

Brooks-Gunn and Ruble (1980) found that both boys and girls in
the seventh and eighth grades have similar and mostly negative
beliefs about menstruation. For example, most believed that menstruation is accompanied by physical discomfort, increased emotionality, and a disruption of activities. Only a third thought that the
onset of menstruation was something to be happy about.

Williams (1983) found more positive attitudes toward menstruation in a group of 9 to 12 year old girls, most of whom were
premenarcheal. These girls generally equated menstruation with
growing up and being normal. However, about a third of these subjects also believed menstruation to be embarassing, 28 percent
thought it a nuisance, 27 percent found it disgusting, and 23 percent
disliked the idea that it is not controllable. The girls in this sample
also believed some of the popular menstrual taboos. About half the
subjects thought a girl should not swim when menstruating and 22
percent believed she should not be active in sports. Many were influenced by concealment taboos with a majority expressing concern
about concealing sanitary pads and menstrual odor. A striking 85
percent thought that a girl should not talk about menstruation to boys
and 40 percent did not even think that it was all right to discuss

menstruation with their fathers. And, as in the Brooks-Gunn and Ruble study noted above, most believed that girls are more emotional when they menstruate.

Reactions to Menarche

What do girls actually experience at the time of menarche? In several studies menarche has been found to be an anxiety producing or negative event (Brooks-Gunn & Ruble, 1980; Golub & Catalano, 1983; Koff, Rierdan, & Jacobson, 1981; Whisnant & Zegans, 1975) and mixed feelings such as being "excited but scared" or "happy and embarrassed" are common (Petersen, 1983; Woods, Dery, & Most, 1983). Most of these data were collected using interviews and questionnaires, and sometimes were based on recollections of older subjects.

Petersen (1983) in looking at menarche as one part of her study of 400 middle-class suburban boys and girls in the 6th, 7th, and 8th grades, found that the adolescents were remarkably inarticulate in describing their feelings about their changing bodies. Therefore, she decided that projective measures might be more useful than direct questions in exploring girls' feelings about menstruation. The girls were presented with an incomplete story about menarche adapted from Judy Blume's book, *Are You There, God? It's Me, Margaret.* For example:

> "Mom—hey, Mom—come quick!" When Nancy's mother got to the bathroom she said: "What is it? What's the matter?" "I got it," Nancy told her. "Got what?" said her mother.

The girls were then asked, "What happened next?" Some of the girls responded that, "She told her Mom that she had gotten her period;" others said that Mom explained or helped. They were then asked "How did Nancy feel?" About a third gave negative or fearful responses, about half were positive or pleased, and another five percent were ambivalent.

Maxine Kumin (1982) in a short story entitled "Facts of Life" differentiates between the expectations about menarche and its actual occurrence. She describes a group of twelve-year-old girls as longing to begin to menstruate. "An eager band of little girls, itchy with the work of sprouting, sits expectant. The old reticences, embarrassments, and complaints have given way to progress. Now we have sex education, cartoon films of the reproductive tract, a belt-less sanitary napkin, a slender, virginal tampon'' (p. 11). Yet, when the first blood does indeed come the girl is described as both terribly happy and terribly sad as mother and daughter celebrate together.

Changes in Body Image

Changes in body image are among the most dramatic reactions to menarche. Although the body changes associated with puberty occur gradually, girls do expect to act differently after menarche and they also see themselves differently. In a clever study of seventh grade girls, Koff (1983) asked the subjects to draw male and female human figures on two occasions, approximately six months apart. Of the 87 girls sampled, 34 were premenarcheal on both test occasions, 23 were postmenarcheal, and 30 changed menarcheal status between the two test sessions. The findings were striking. Postmenarcheal girls produced drawings that were significantly more sexually differentiated than those of their premenarcheal peers and a greater percentage of the postmenarcheal girls drew their own sex first. Most notable was the difference in the drawings done by the girls whose menarcheal status changed during the course of the study. There was a significant increase in the sexual differentiation of their drawings at the time of the second testing with the postmenarcheal girls drawing womanly females with breasts and curves in contrast to their earlier, more childlike, premenarcheal drawings. (Examples of these drawings may be seen in Koff, 1983.)

To further explore girls' beliefs about the change menarche would have on them, Koff, Rierdan, and Jacobson (1981) gave a sentence completion task to seventh and eighth grade girls. In response to the cue sentence ''Ann just got her period for the first time,'' the girls said such things as, ''She saw herself in a different way,'' and ''She felt very grown up.'' In response to another item, ''Ann regarded her body as . . .,'' postmenarcheal girls were more likely than premenarcheal girls to describe a change in body image. For example, Ann's body was ''a woman's body'' and ''more mature than it was.''

These studies clearly demonstrate that girls do experience menarche as a turning point in their development and they apparently reorganize their body images in the direction of ''greater sexual maturity and feminine differentiation'' (Koff, 1983). Postmenarcheal girls are more aware of sexual differentiation between males and females and of themselves as women than are premenarcheal girls of the same age.

The Early Maturing Girl

The age at which a girl experiences menarche does seem to affect her reaction to it. Peterson (1983) found that girls who experience menarche early, in the sixth grade or before, seem to have more difficulty with it. Some of the girls denied that they had begun to menstruate and when Petersen questioned the mothers of her early maturing subjects, over 70 percent of the mothers reported that menarche was very difficult for their daughters. The mothers of five of the six girls who denied having gotten their periods reported the negative aspects of the experience for them. Notman (1983) has suggested that the denial of menstruation may be related to conflicts about accepting the female role or to an attempt to delay adulthood. Certainly one of the girls in Petersen's sample who denied menstruating lends support to that view. In response to a Thematic Apperception Test card showing a middle-aged woman with a girl holding a doll, this subject described the girl in the picture as scared about growing up and asking her mother when she was going to get her period.

Unlike boys who are eager for their growth spurt and physical signs of maturity, girls would prefer to mature at the same time as everyone else. This may be because of the age difference between the sexes in the onset of puberty—boys normally start later than girls. Girls' attitudes about early development may also be related to the changes in their lives that occur when they develop the breasts and curves characteristic of a woman. There is some evidence that sixth and seventh grade girls who are already pubertal are more likely to be dating and, somewhat paradoxically, these girls also have lower self-esteem, lower school achievement, and more behavioral problems than comparable boys and non-pubertal girls (Simmons, Blyth, Van Cleave, & Bush, 1979). In this study pubertal development per se had little effect on the girls' self-esteem. However, the early maturing girls who had also begun dating were most likely to indicate low self-esteem (50 percent as opposed to 36-40 percent of the other girls). It is interesting that while early dating behavior is disadvantageous for girls, it has no statistically significant impact on boys.

Thus girls' self-esteem was negatively affected by their own physiology (early menarche) and social relationships, while boys' self-esteeem was not. Simons et al. (1979) suggest some reason why this may be so. First, the sexes develop different value systems at this age. For girls, appearance and sociability assume priority, while for boys these values remain secondary. When asked to rank the importance of popularity, competence, and independence, seventh grade girls were more likely to rank popularity first. This places a great deal of importance on other peoples' opinions of oneself. These girls also placed a high value on looks. Moreover, the changes in body image may be qualitatively different for girls than for boys. Pubertal boys are generally happy with their new height and muscle development. Pubertal girls are not sure whether their new figures make them better or worse looking than their peers. Further, pubertal girls' negative reactions to dating may be a result of sexual pressures from their male partners for which these girls are not prepared. In interviews with some of these girls the researchers found them likely to express dislike for "guys trying to touch me." One subject said, "I don't really like to be kissed." It looks as if some of these girls were vulnerable, with their emotional maturity lagging well behind their physical development, causing confusion and contributing to their feelings of low self-esteem. This is in keeping with data from the California Adolescent Study which show that it is the girl with accelerated growth and maturation who is at a disadvantage (Jones, 1958; Jones & Mussen, 1959). However, social class may also play a role. Clausen (1975) found that for middle-class girls' early maturation was positively related to self-confidence, whereas working class girls experienced a negative effect. In contrast to early maturation, late maturation, although quite disturbing for boys, does not seem to have the same degree of negative consequences for girls, perhaps because a childlike appearance is part of femininity for some adult women (Friedman, Note 2).

Relationships with Parents

In view of the changes that go on in girls' perceptions of themselves it seems reasonable to ask if menarche affects girls' relationships with other people, particularly family members. On the basis of limited data, the answer seems to be a qualified yes. Danza (1983) compared 48 pre- and postmenarcheal girls in the sixth and seventh grades. She found that although they were no different in age than their premenarcheal peers, the postmenarcheal girls were more likely to wear make-up or a bra, to shave their legs, and to date. They also slept less on school nights, moving from nine or more hours a night toward the more usual adult eight hour sleep cycle. The postmenarcheal girls were also significantly more uncomfortable in discussing emotionally charged topics such as love, sex, drugs, and alcohol with their parents, and they reported having more conflict with their parents than the premenarcheal girls did.

Effects on Sexual Behavior

Because it marks the onset of reproductive potential, menarche is important to a girl's family and community as well as to herself. This is seen in other cultures when one looks at the different tribal rituals celebrating menarche and at customs, such as purdah, veiling, and virginity tests, which guard girls' reproductive potential. Economics comes into play too. Paige (1983) has suggested that there is a relationship between various methods of controlling girls' chastity and the economic resources of a particular culture. In societies where marriage bargains are important, chastity is crucial to the girl's marriageability and is rigorously controlled.

This is not seen in our culture today. Rather, in the United States the physical transformation from girl to woman and the onset of menstruation are accompanied by changes in social and sexual behavior. And the timing of menarche is important. Several researchers have reported that girls with an early menarche were more likely to date and pet at an earlier age than their later maturing peers (Gagnon, 1983; Presser, 1978; Simons et al., 1979; Udry, 1979). And there is data indicating that women with early menarche begin premarital coitus earlier as well (Gagnon, 1983; Presser, 1978; Udry, 1979). In an extensive study of black and white low income women in 16 American cities, Udry (1979) found that girls with early menarche, as compared to those with late menarche, were more than twice as likely to have had intercourse by age 16. Udry and Cliquet (1982) also examined the relationship between ages at menarche, marriage, and first birth among women in four widely diverse countries (United States, Malay, Belgium, and Pakistan) and concluded that there was a clear behavioral sequence relating age at menarche to age at first intercourse and first birth. Menarche seems to initiate a chain of events. In the United States the pattern is one of dating and other sexual behavior that increase the probability of early intercourse and early childbearing.

Whether this sequence is more readily attributable to hormonal or sociocultural factors is a difficult question to answer. Gagnon (1983) found no significant relationship between the onset of menarche and masturbatory experience. Similarly, in their studies of children with the problem of precocious puberty (beginning at six to eight years of age), Ehrhardt and Meyer-Bahlberg (1975) have found that early puberty does not automatically trigger an early sex life. Masturbation and sex play in childhood did not appear to be enhanced and premarital intercourse did not occur earlier than normally expected. Thus at this time it seems reasonable to conclude that the timing of puberty influences when the girl, her parents, and her peers perceive of her as being someone for whom dating and heterosexual relationships are appropriate and this in turn affects her socio-sexual behavior.

Preparation of Menarche

In view of the ambivalent feelings about menarche expressed by so many adolescent girls and the difficulties experienced by the early maturing girl, it seems reasonable to ask if adequate preparation makes any difference? It probably does. Both Rierdan (1983) and Golub and Catalano (1983) found that subjects who report being adequately prepared have a more positive initial experience with menstruation. There are other studies indicating a need for more and better menstrual education. For example, Logan (1980), in a study of 95 women from 23 foreign countries, found that 28 percent complained about not having enough information. Similarly, in a large study of American women, 39 percent reported that their preparation was inadequate (Weideger, 1976). And Brooks-Gunn and Ruble (1980) reported that the adolescent girls they tested said they had sufficient prior knowledge about menstruation but still felt unprepared for menarche.

What do girls want to know? Rierdan (1983), in a study of 97 college women's recollections of menarche, found that the young women wanted to know about menstrual physiology and menstrual hygiene—the facts that are usually included in menstrual education materials—but they also wanted information about menstruation as a personal event. Subjects said that girls need to know about the normality of menstruation and it must be distinguished from disease, injury, and uncleanliness. They suggested that the feelings of fright and embarrassment girls experience at menarche be acknowledged as normal and the negative aspects of the menstrual experience need to be discussed in order to provide a balanced view of menstruation. The college women emphasized that girls need support and reassurance at the time of menarche and Rierdan says, "Many referred specifically to the importance of an informed, understanding, accepting mother" (Rierdan, 1983). Unfortunately, however, interviews with mothers of adolescent girls indicate that the mothers themselves are not prepared to fill this role, suggesting a need to prepare mothers as well as daughters for menarche.

In Support of a New Tradition

Some researchers have suggested that we need a "contemporary tradition for menarche" in order to overcome some of the negative connotations associated with it (Logan, Calder, & Cohen, 1980). They believe that currently we address the physical needs of the menarcheal girl, teaching her how to take care of herself, but leaving her without the social and emotional support that she needs at this time. In order to explore what the appropriate ritual might be, Logan et al. designed five short stories describing possible responses to a girl's first period and gave them to girls between the ages of eight and seventeen, mothers of girls in this age group, and women psychologists. The most popular response of the mothers and daughters to being told about the onset of menstruation was "Congratulations, our little girl is growing up." However, the psychologists preferred, "Something special has happened," apparently acknowledging the ambivalent and even negative emotions that a girl may have about the beginning of menstruation. As for symbolic gestures, the most popular among the mothers was a toast to the girl from her mother and father, or a meal in her honor. But the daughters had reservations about this, fearing an invasion of privacy and reinforcing feelings that "everyone is watching her." The daughters preferred a hug or a kiss and a material token such as a gift or flowers. It seems dramatists often capture in a few lines what scientists seek in reams of data: William Alfred was right on target with the gift of a brooch.

REFERENCE NOTES

1. Menkin, J., Watkins, S. C., & Trussell, J. Nutrition, health, and fertility. Report prepared for The Ford Foundation. December 1980.

2. Freedman, R. Personal Communication. December 1983.

REFERENCES

Benedek, T. Sexual functions in women and their disturbance. In S. Arieti (Ed.) *American handbook of psychiatry.* New York: Basic Books, 1959.

Blume, J. *Are you there, God? It's me, Margaret.* New York: Dell, 1970.

Brennock, W. E. Fertility at menarche. *Medical Aspects of Human Sexuality,* 1982, *16,* 21-30.

Brooks-Gunn, J., & Ruble, D. Menarche. In A. J. Dan, E. A. Graham, & C. P. Beecher (Eds.) *The menstrual cycle. Vol. 1.* New York: Springer, 1980.

Chern, M. M., Gatewood, L. C., & Anderson, V. E. The inheritance of menstrual traits. In A. J. Dan, E. A. Graham, & C. P. Beecher (Eds.) *The menstrual cycle. Vol. 1.* New York: Springer, 1980

Clausen, J. A. The social meaning of differential physical and sexual maturation. In S. E. Dragastin, & G. H. Elder, Jr. (Eds.) *Adolescence in the life cycle.* New York: Halsted, 1975.

Danza, R. Menarche: Its effects on mother-daughter and father-daughter interactions. In S. Golub (Ed.) *Menarche.* Lexington, Massachusetts: D. C. Heath, 1983.

Dupon, C. & Bingel, A. S. Endocrinologic changes associated with puberty in girls. In A. J. Dan, E. A. Graham, & C. P. Beecher (Eds.) *The menstrual cycle. Vol. 1* New York: Springer, 1980.

Ehrhardt, A. E., & Meyer-Bahlberg, H. F. L. Psychological correlates of abnormal pubertal development. *Clinics in Endocrinology and Metabolism.* 1975, *4,* 207-222.

Ellison, P. T. Skeletal growth, fatness, and menarcheal age: A comparison of two hypotheses. *Human Biology,* 1982, *54,* 269-281.

Freud, A. *The ego and the mechanisms of defense.* New York: International Universities Press, 1946.

Frisch, R. E. Fatness, puberty and fertility. *Natural History,* 1980, *89,* 16-27.

Frisch, R. E. What's below the surface. *New England Journal of Medicine,* 1981, *305,* 1019-1020.

Frisch, R. E., Gotz-Welbergen, A. V., McArthur, J. W., Albright, T., Witschi, J., Bullen, B., Birnholz, J., Reed, R.B., & Hermann, H. Delayed menarche and amenorrhea of college athletes in relation to age of onset of training. *Journal of the American Medical Association,* 1981, *246,* 1559-1563.

Frisch, R. E. Fatness, menarche, and fertility. In S. Golub (Ed.) *Menarche.* Lexington, Massachusetts: D. C. Heath, 1983.

Gagnon, J. H. Age at menarche and sexual conduct in adolescence and young adulthood. In S. Golub (Ed.) *Menarche.* Lexington, Massachusetts: D. C. Heath, 1983.

Golub, S., & Catalano, J. Recollections of menarche and women's subsequent experiences with menstruation. *Women & Health,* 1983, *8,* 49-61.

Goodman, M. J., Grove, J. S., & Gilbert, R. I. Age at menarche and year of birth in relation to adult height and weight among Caucasian, Japanese and Chinese women living in Hawaii. In S. Golub (Ed.) *Menarche.* Lexington, Massachusetts, D. C. Heath, 1983.

Grumbach, M. M, Grave, G. D., & Mayer, F. E. (Eds.) *Control of the onset of puberty.* New York: Wiley, 1974.

Jones, M. C. A study of socialization patterns at the high school level. *Journal of Genetic Psychology,* 1958, *93,* 87-111.

Jones, M. C., & Mussen, P. H. Self conceptions, motivations, and interpersonal attitudes of early and late maturing girls. *Child Development,* 1958, *29,* 491-501.

Kantero, R. L., & Widholm, O. Correlation of menstrual traits between adolescent girls and their mothers. *Acta Obstetricia et Gynecologica Scandinavica, Supplement,* 1971, *14,* 30-36.

Katchadourian, H. The biology of adolescence. San Francisco: W. H. Freeman & Co., 1977.

Kestenberg, J. S. Menarche. In S. Lorand, & H. Schneer (Eds.) *Adolescents.* New York: Dell, 1965.

Koff, E., Rierdan, J., & Silverstone, E. Changes in representation of body image as a function of menarcheal status. *Developmental Psychology,* 1978, *14,* 635-642.

Koff, E., Rierdan, J., & Jacobson, S. The personal and interpersonal significance of menarche. *Journal of the American Academy of Child Psychiatry,* 1981, *20,* 148-158.

Koff, E. Through the looking glass of menarche: What the adolescent girl sees. In S. Golub (Ed.) *Menarche.* Lexington, Massachusetts, D. C. Heath, 1983.

Kumin, M. *Why can't we live together like civilized human beings?* New York: Viking Press, 1982.

Leppert, P. Menarche and adolescent pregnancy. In S. Golub (Ed.) *Menarche.* Lexington, Massachusetts: D. C. Heath, 1983.

Logan, D. D. The menarche experience in twenty-three foreign countries. *Adolescence,* 1980, *15,* 247-256.

Malina, R. M. Delayed age of menarche of athletes. *Journal of the American Medical Association,* 1982, *247,* 3312.

Notman, M. Menarche: A psychoanalytic perspective. In S. Golub (Ed.) *Menarche.* Lexington, Massachusetts: D. C. Heath, 1983.

Paige, K. E. Virginity rituals and chastity control during puberty: Cross-cultural patterns. In S. Golub (Ed.) *Menarche.* Lexington, Massachusetts: D. C. Heath, 1983.

Petersen, A. C., & Taylor, B. The biological approach to adolescence. In J. Adelson (Ed.) *Handbook of adolescent psychology.* New York: Wiley, 1980.

Petersen, A. E. Menarche: Meaning of measures and measuring meaning. In S. Golub (Ed.) *Menarche.* Lexington, Massachusetts: D. C. Heath, 1983.

Presser, H. B. Age at menarche, socio-sexual behavior, and fertility. *Social Biology,* 1978, *25,* 94-101.

Rebar, R. W., & Cumming, D. C. Reproductive function in women athletes. *Journal of the American Medical Association,* 1981, *246,* 1590.

Rierdan, J. Variations in the experience of menarche as a function of preparedness. In S. Golub (Ed.) *Menarche.* Lexington, Massachusetts: D. C. Heath, 1983.

Rosenbaum, M. B. The changing body image of the adolescent girl. In M. Sugar (Ed.) *Female adolescent development.* New York: Brunner/Mazel, 1979.

Shields, J. *Monozygotic twins.* London: Oxford University Press, 1962.

Simmons, R. G., Blyth, D. A., Van Cleave, E. F., & Bush, D. M. Entry into early adolescence: The impact of school structure, puberty, and early dating on self esteem. *American Sociological Review,* 1979, *44,* 948-967.

Tanner, J. M. *Foetus into man.* Cambridge, Massachusetts: Harvard University Press, 1978.

To everything there is a season. *Science News,* 1980, *118,* 150.

Udry, J. R. Age at menarche, at first intercourse, and at first pregnancy. *Journal of Biosocial Science,* 1979, *11,* 433-441.

Udry, J. R., & Cliquet, R. L. A cross-cultural examination of the relationship between ages at menarche, marriage, and first birth. *Demography,* 1982, *19,* 53-63.

Warren, M. P. Clinical aspects of menarche: Normal variations and common disorders. In S. Golub (Ed.) *Menarche.* Lexington, Massachusetts: D. C. Heath, 1983.

Weideger, P. *Menstruation and menopause.* New York: Knopf, 1976.

Whisnant, L., & Zegans, L. A study of attitudes toward menarche in white middle class American adolescent girls. *American Journal of Psychiatry,* 1975, *132,* 809-814.

Williams, L. R. Beliefs and attitudes of young girls regarding menstruation. In S. Golub (Ed.) *Menarche.* Lexington, Massachusetts: D. C. Heath, 1983.

Woods, N. F., Dery, G. K., & Most, A. Recollections of menarche, current menstrual attitudes, and perimenstrual symptoms. In S. Golub (Ed.) *Menarche.* Lexington, Massachusetts: D. C. Heath, 1983.

Menstrual Health Products, Practices, and Problems

Nancy Reame, RN, PhD

ABSTRACT. This review article examines factors affecting normal variations in menstrual flow, methods used to estimate vaginal blood loss, menstrual health problems related to hygiene practices, and methods of assessing tampon absorbancy. Preliminary studies from this laboratory suggest that normal, cycling women exhibit menstrual flow rates that are significantly higher during the day than at night; also that menstrual blood has a more acid pH than previously reported, and that it demonstrates unique biological properties unlike peripheral venous blood. Women in wheelchairs may be at special risk for the development of menstrual health problems because of difficulties with hygiene management as evidenced by results of a study of 22 women with traumatic spinal cord injuries.

As long as women have been menstruating, there has been a need for a safe, effective, convenient, and comfortable way of managing menstrual flow. Regardless of shape, size, or composition, menstrual hygiene products have for centuries been one of two varieties: internal or external. It has only been within the last 60 years that these products have been made commercially and only since 1980 with their reported association with toxic shock syndrome that they have come under medical, political, and public scrutiny (Shands et al. 1980). With this scrutiny has come the realization that very little research (outside of closely guarded in-house studies by the tampon industry) has been focused on the physiology of menstruation, the dynamics of menstrual flow and product absorbancy, and health problems associated with menstrual hygiene. As recently as 1978, a survey by Consumer Reports of 4500 users of menstrual tampons and pads reported that "some women were worried that tampons could lead to vaginal or bladder infection, to erosion of the cervix, to hemorrhaging or to uterine growths . . . But our medical consultants assured us that neither tampons or pads are a hazard to

37

health . . . .Some women occasionally forget to remove a tampon and notice a bad odor or discharge a week or so later. But that condition is not serious. Symptoms usually disappear soon after the tampon is removed.''

In 1980, the Food and Drug Administration (FDA) adopted a rule classifying menstrual tampons under the Medical Device Amendments of 1976 as class II medical devices. For thirty years, tampons and pads had been classified as cosmetics and had only recently been upgraded to the general category of "devices." An effect of this new classification was to provide for the development of a national performance standard for the safety and efficacy of menstrual tampons. (Menstrual pads are classified as class I medical devices being in the same category as tongue depressors and therefore are not subject to performance standards.) To establish a standard for tampon performance, disclosure of ingredients, and labeling requirements, the FDA approached the national organization that develops voluntary manufacturing standards for all commercially produced materials and goods, the American Society for Testing of Materials (ASTM). ASTM responded by creating a task force of interested tampon producers (Kimberly-Clark Corp., Tampax Corp., Personal Products Corp., Playtex Corp., Johnson and Johnson), consumer groups, and FDA members to develop such a standard (Cohen, 1982). The charge of the task force may seem straightforward, but in order to determine minimum standards and tests for absorbancy, biocompatability, sterility, and method and duration of use implies an understanding of menstruation that may be as yet only theoretical. The purpose of this paper will be to review current knowledge of menstrual function as well as to describe preliminary clinical and laboratory studies designed to better define normal menstrual health.

MENSTRUAL BLOOD: COMPOSITION AND VOLUME OF FLOW

To develop the perfect tampon requires that it be designed to optimally interact with the appropriate fluid. The classic text book description of menstrual exudate as a composition of blood, mucus, cellular debris, and bacteria is based on the studies that date back to the turn of the century when the cytology, hemotology, and biochemistry of menstrual secretions were first examined in an ef-

fort to determine its diagnostic value in infertility and other gynecologic disease (Barer & Fowler, 1936; Champneys, 1891; Stickel &
Zondek, 1920). In the 1940s significant interest was raised about a
menstrual toxin which according to the investigators was specific to
the menstrual serum, present in high concentrations in the endometrial cells, and was lethal to young rats within 48 hours after a
single injection (Smith & Smith, 1945). They hypothesized that
menstruation was a toxic phenomenon meant to rid the body of
poisons. Macht(1943) had found in the sweat, saliva, and circulating
blood of menstruating women a substance which he claimed was
toxic to plant growth. Work in the '50s refuted these studies by
showing that lab animals who died after the injection of menstrual
toxin were found to have a bacterial infection as a result of contamination of the samples due to poor laboratory technique (Zondek,
1953). Later studies have focused on the fluidity of menstrual fluid
and the mechanism of clotting and fibrinolysis (Beller, 1971;
Christiaens et al., 1981; Ebert, et al., 1979). A variety of clinical
and laboratory methods have been used to assess menstrual fluid
characteristics. Samples have been collected by curettage, in
vaginal/cervical cups, at hysterectomy, by tampons, by aspiration at
the time of IUD insertion and even by intravaginal placement of a
glass tube while the women remained in bed for the duration of their
periods (Beller, 1971; Burnhill & Birnberg, 1965; Christiaens et
al., 1981; Couture, Freund, & Sedlis, 1979; Geist, 1929).

As reviewed by Beller & Schweppe, (1979), a variety of organic
compounds, minerals and hormones have been identified in
menstrual fluid. Prostaglandin F, the hormone-like substance which
stimulates painful muscle contractions, has been found in high concentrations in the menstrual discharge of women who suffer from
severe menstrual cramps (Pickles et al, 1965). Significant iron loss
in the menses has been associated with low venous values of
hemoglobin and hematocrit in anemic women (Rybo, 1966). The
pH of menstrual fluid has been reported to be alkaline, ranging between 6.9 and 7.5 (Bussing, 1957; Ebert et al., 1979). Menstrual
blood has been shown to be more viscous than peripheral venous
blood (Bussing, 1957). Few of these biochemical parameters have
been evaluated to see how they change throughout the menstrual
period or from cycle to cycle and woman to woman. Several of
these studies determined values on pooled samples collected from a
number of women across different days of menses.

One of the problems associated with setting a tampon performance standard is determining the normal amount of menstrual blood loss. Most investigators agree that there is a dramatic variation among women in the nature and amount of monthly flow although the average menstrual blood loss is considered to be 30 ml (about 2 fluid ounces) and the average flow of 4 days duration (Hallberg & Nilsson, 1964; Shaw, Aaronson, & Moyer, 1972). Several factors have been examined to explain variations in menstrual flow characteristics among women. The most commonly considered variables for assessment are age and parity. In a study of 476 Swedish women, six age groups between 15 and 50 years were sampled (Hallberg et al., 1966). Females in the youngest and oldest groups had significantly different blood losses, but within the age range of 23 to 45 years, age had no influence.

Several investigators have observed no significant influence of parity on blood loss (Hallberg & Nilsson, 1964; Hytten, Cheyne, & Klopper, 1964), while others have reported that "ever-pregnant" women have heavier blood losses than "never-pregnant" women of the same age group (Barer & Fowler, 1936; Cole, Billewicz, & Thomson, 1971). Parity does not appear to be a significant factor in the etiology of menorrhagia, or prolonged menstrual bleeding (Haynes et al., 1977). There is little evidence for a long-term effect of induced abortion on duration of menses (Andreev, 1970). Cole et al., (1971) have shown that menstrual blood loss is related to parity, subject's height, and birthweight of offspring, suggesting that uterine size is an important factor in relation to amount of flow. However, they were unable to explain the wide range of blood loss that still persisted in women of the same age, stature, and parity. Rybo (1966) reported that birthweight of children did not affect total menstrual blood loss.

Other factors that have been reported as sources of variation in menstrual blood loss among healthy women include heredity, length of menses, and menstrual symptoms. The average menstrual blood loss appears similar among contempory Swedish, US, English, and Egyptian populations (Hallberg & Nilsson, 1964; Hefnawi et al., 1977; Hytten et al., 1964; Shaw et al., 1972), but Ober (1952) reported that women of primitive tribes experience a total menstrual period of a few drops and lasting half an hour. In a study of monozygotic and dizygotic pairs of twins, hereditary factors were show to influence volume of blood loss (Rybo, 1966). Since most studies have deliberately selected homogeneous populations for examination, ethnic variability as it exists in contemporary American society has not been adequately explored. The occurrence of dysmenorrhea or appearance of clots in the discharge are not necessarily associated with heavy flow (Stevenson et al., 1945). Conflicting reports exist with respect to a positive correlation between duration of menses and total menstrual blood loss (Haynes et al., 1977; Rybo, 1966; Stevenson et al., 1945).

Pattern of menstrual flow has been studied primarily in relation to daily menstrual blood loss. The majority of menstrual bleeding occurs during the first two days in both eumenorrheic and menorrhagic women (Haynes et al., 1977). Menstrual blood appears to be expelled forcefully from the cervix in sporadic episodes and may exhibit different flow rates depending on the hour and day of menstruation (Hinselmann, 1925).

Little information is available on differences between night and day patterns of flow. In a study involving 84 nursing students in 1945, 58% began menstruating in the morning, 19% in the afternoon, and 22% during the night (Stevenson et al., 1945). The time of onset of successive periods was approximately the same. The effect of work shift or sleeping habits on time of onset or patterns of flow was not examined.

The type of occupation may also influence menstrual flow characteristics. Although menstrual cycle irregularity, amount of discharge, and dysmenorrheic symptoms have been reported to increase among airline flight attendants flying across time zones, it is not known whether these effects are due to change in activity level, sleep deprivation, light-dark cycle, altitude, endocrine biorhythms, or stress in general (Preston et al., 1974). An increased incidence of hypomenorrhea and oligomenorrhea among female athletes is believed due to a change in critical body mass and the ratio between lean muscle to fat (Frisch, 1983).

Oral contraceptives and the IUD are known to significantly affect the degree and/or nature of menstrual blood loss. The combination and low-dose types of birth control pills have been associated with lighter and shorter pseudo-menses. Both the copper and progestogen-containing IUD are associated with less menstrual blood loss and cramping than the inert types (Tatum, 1973). Because progestogens increase the viscosity of cervical mucus and copper-bearing IUDs decrease cervical mucus viscosity, the use of contraceptives may affect the fluidity of the menstrual fluid and ultimately product absorbancy (Jeffcoate, 1975). Although duration of flow and total blood loss is similar during ovulatory and anovulatory cycles, mucin content as well as other properties of menstrual fluid may be altered when hormonal influence is minimal (Poon et al., 1973).

Since quantitation of vaginal bleeding has direct clinical application, several techniques have been developed to estimate menstrual blood loss. The traditional method is to ask women to report the number of days of menstrual bleeding or the number of tampons or pads used as a function of time. As referred to previously, duration of flow may bear little relation to the total volume (Barer & Fowler, 1938; Hytten et al., 1964). Estimating blood loss by pad or tampon use is based on the assumption that the amount of blood absorbed by different types and brands is known and equivalent. Although one source suggested that both pads and tampons will absorb 20 to 30 ml of blood when totally saturated, another reference reported that completely wet pads absorb approximately 50 ml more menstrual blood than tampons (Schnatz, 1975; Beller & Schweepe, 1979). Grimes (1979) conducted a study of absorption capacities of 15 types of menstrual napkins, pads, and tampons using a device that dropped venous blood obtained from a hospital blood bank onto the central surface of each product at a constant rate of 2.47 ml per minute. There was significant variation in absorption abilities among the products tested, with some napkins absorbing nearly 5 times more fluid than some tampon brands. Products from the same package showed substantial variation in amounts of blood absorbed. The investigator inferred from this laboratory assessment that estimating blood loss by counting the number of products worn is unlikely to yield reliable information.

Another method that has been used to determine quantity of blood loss is to have women collect all pre-weighed menstrual tampons or pads used during an entire period in airtight containers to avoid evaporation and then weigh them again after use, giving an estimate of menstrual discharge in grams of wet weight (Stevenson et al., 1945). The alkaline hematin method has been used widely and measures the amount of hemoglobin breakdown product by means of a colorimetric test that is present in a used product. The blood volume is then calculated by a conversion formula which assumes that the hemoglobin of menstrual blood approximates that of peripheral venous blood (Newton, Barnard, & Collines, 1977; Shaw et al., 1972). As reviewed by Beller and Schweppe (1979), several investigators have described hemoglobin and hematocrit values for menstrual blood far below those for venous blood. A study supported by Johnson and Johnson Co. estimated menstrual volume by collecting menses in a rubber intra-vaginal cup for direct measurement of ml of fluid (Schmidt, 1966). The researchers noted that with practice, spillage during removal was minimal. Methods that estimate gross volume or weight of menstrual material may better reflect the contribution of other components such as cells and mucus to the discharge in addition to blood.

Several clinical and laboratory studies have been performed by this investigator to better define normal menstrual health as well as to identify women who might be at special risk for menstrual health problems (Reame, Note 2; Reame, Note 3; Reame, Note 4; Reame, Note 5). In 1977, three years before toxic shock syndrome became a household phrase, a study was initiated at the request of Kimberly-Clark Corporation, makers of Kotex products, to examine the contents and flow characteristics of menstrual fluid as a preliminary step in the development of a comparable synthetic vaginal fluid that could be used for testing product absorbancy. Most tampon makers use some type of "syngyna fluid" in their laboratory studies (Friedman, 1981). A recipe for the syngyna fluid used by the FDA is presented in Table 1.

Over an 18-month period, 122 samples of menstrual fluid were collected from 27 women during 58 cycles. Subjects were recruited from a population of healthy, urban hospital employees and selected on the basis of negative gynecologic exam findings, normal menstrual history, and the use of a contraceptive method other than the birth control pill or IUD. Samples were collected by means of an

Table 1. "Syngyna Fluid:" A Synthetic Menses Fluid
          Used by the Center for Medical Device Analysis,
          Food and Drug Administration, for Testing Tampon
          Absorbancy. *

Components	Amount (grams)
Sodium chloride	10.0
Sodium bicarbonate	4.0
Cellulose Gum	4.0
Glycerol	100.0
Water	880.0
Food Coloring	trace

* Marlowe, D.E., Weigle, R.M., Stauffengerg, R.S. Measurement of
  Tampon Absorbancy - Test Method Evaluation. CMDA Report 81-013,
  May, 1981. Bureau of Medical Devices, FDA, 8757 Georgia Avenue,
  Silver Spring, MD 20910

intravaginal rubber menstrual cup which had been sold commercially as an over-the-counter product by Tassette, Inc. until 1972 as an alternative to tampons (Pena, 1962). Women were instructed on the insertion and removal of the cup and allowed to practice its use prior to wearing them for study. An estimate of flow rate was determined by dividing sample volumes by the number of insertion hours. Menstrual flow rates of samples collected during the day were more than two times higher than for those samples collected on an overnight basis while subjects were sleeping. Age, parity, weight, height, incidence of cramps, and time of bleeding onset did not significantly influence menstrual flow volumes. The finding that flow rate has a significant diurnal variation suggests that product needs of menstruating women at night (i.e., while asleep) may be different from daytime needs and that further study is needed of such possible influences as level of activity, metabolic rate, and peripheral blood flow.

The viscosity of menstrual fluid was examined in 25 samples during 14 cycles from 10 women using a Wells-Brookefield microviscometer. This study revealed that menstrual fluid was more viscous when compared to venous blood even though it had a much lower hematocrit (which in peripheral blood is the primary influence on viscosity). In addition, the viscosity of menstrual fluid was highest on the first day of menses and gradually dropped with subsequent days of flow. Menstrual discharge behaved in terms of viscosity more like an oil-based paint, having small particles suspended in a thick fluid. This finding suggests that the fluid of choice for the conduct of tampon/pad absorbancy testing may not be peripheral venous blood which has been used in some studies (Reingold, Note 6; 1982. Shaw et al., 1972) The contribution of other fluids to the "thickness" of menstrual exudate such as cervical mucus or vaginal secretions needs further study.

Sixty-three specimens of menstrual fluid from 10 women were examined for pH. Although the mean pH of all samples was 6.3, there was a wide range in values which was statistically significant for subject variation (p = .01). The mean pH for subjects ranged from 4.7 to 7.3. This subject-specific relationship was not influenced by time of collection, duration of wear, or day of menses. Flow rate was found to be the only factor that significantly influenced the pH: the faster the rate of flow, the higher the pH. Those subjects with a mean pH in the alkaline range (above 7.0 had a significantly higher (faster) rate of menstrual flow. This phenomenon can perhaps be explained on the basis of length of in utero degradation of menstrual blood products. Those specimens associated with slow rates of flow perhaps experienced greater lysis of red blood cells and tissue resulting in release of their highly acid, internal constituents. An example of differences in mean flow rates and pH of menstrual specimens between two normal subjects followed for 3 consecutive cycles is presented in Table 2.

In order to determine the importance of differences in menstrual fluid pH on the vaginal environment, an in vitro study was undertaken of the ability of menstrual fluid to serve as a vehicle for sperm transport, (Reame, Note 3). Much is known about the pH requirements for optimum motility and survivability of sperm in the female reproductive tract (Vander Vliet & Hafez, 1974). A hostile cervical mucus with a pH outside the normal range of 7.0 to 8.5 has been identified as a cause of subfertility in women (Moghissi, 1979). Fifty specimens of menstrual fluid obtained from 10 healthy women were tested for penetrability and spermicidal effects on semen samples collected from fertile donors with sperm counts of at least 60 million/ml. The two fluids were placed on a microscope slide, covered, and examined at the point of interface using a light microscope. The number of live motile sperm was assessed in successive high power fields at timed intervals as recommended by Moghissi and Syner (1970) for the clinical evaluation of sperm-mucus interactions. The degree of viability was significantly correlated with the pH of the menstrual fluid ($p = .05$). Samples exhibiting zero viability at 15 minutes or less had a mean pre-test pH of 5.04 compared to a mean pH of 6.6 for those with zero viability at 1 to 5 hours. These findings suggest that women with typically acid flows may be

Table 2. Mean flow rates and pH of menstrual fluid specimens collected from 2 normal women during 3 consecutive cycles.

		DAY OF MENSES		
		Day 1	Day 2	Day 3
Subject A	Flow Rate (ml/hr)	0.5	0.5	0.2
Subject B		2.0	2.0	3.3
Subject A	pH	5.3	6.6	5.0
Subject B		7.4	7.2	7.2

at less risk for invasion by organisms requiring an alkaline environment.

TAMPONS AND VAGINAL HEALTH

Menstrual hygiene practices have been linked to a variety of vaginal health problems including ulcerations, intermenstrual spotting, abnormal discharge, urinary stress incontinence, and toxic shock syndrome (Friedrich, 1981). Friedrich and Siegesmund (1980) demonstrated that microulcerations of the vagina were associated with tampon use especially of the superabsorbant type and when worn for reasons other than to manage menstrual flow. Vaginal lacerations causing serious hemorrhage have been attributed to plastic tampon inserters (Collins, 1979). The incidence of tampon use continuously (day and night) during the menstrual period is significantly greater among toxic shock victims than for matched controls (Shands et al., 1980). Although the duration of tampon wear has not been linked to a higher risk of toxic shock syndrome (TSS), it has been suggested that too frequent changing may lead to pathologic changes of the vaginal mucosa (Davis et al., 1980). Others have speculated that prolonged wear may increase the likelihood of a tampon to act as a culture medium for pathologic organisms (Shands et al., 1980). Probably the strongest evidence linking toxic shock syndrome with menstrual hygiene practices was showing an 8 fold greater incidence of TSS in users of the super absorbant tampon Rely which resulted in its withdrawal from the market in 1980 by its manufacturer, Procter and Gamble Co. (MMWR, 1980). Since that time all major tampon brands have been associated with toxic shock to the extent that the Institute of Medicine issued a strong warning against the use of all high absorbancy, ''super-plus'' tampons especially by young women aged 15 to 24 years (Sun, 1982).

It is not known why Rely tampons were so clearly linked to the etiology of TSS. Enhanced absorbancy, longer duration of wear, differences in chemical additives have been suggested as possible causes for its role in toxic shock (Friedman, 1981). When examined by the scanning electron microscope, an instrument which magnifies surfaces up to 100,000 times, there are dramatic differences in the architecture of Rely before and after use when compared with other more traditional tampon brands (Reame, Note 4). The polyester mini-sponges, which together with superabsorbant cellulose particles are loosely encased in Rely's polyester flow-through sack, exhibited massive surface coating with red blood cells after four hours of tampon wear on the first day of menstrual flow. Specimens from other tampon brands displayed coating of their surfaces with vaginal cells forming an effective barrier to red blood cell penetration into deeper fiber layers. These differences in absorbancy characteristics require further study before a plausible etiologic explanation is clear.

Other investigators have performed comparative studies of absorbancy differences among various tampon brands. Using a "syngyna," an instrument that is said to replicate intra-vaginal pressures, temperature, size, and shape, Osterholm has shown that Playtex regular is more absorbant than Tampax regular and equal in absorbancy to Johnson and Johnson's O.B. super (Sun, 1982). Such discrepancies between product labels and actual tampon performance indicate the need for a standardized absorbancy test against which all brands can be comparatively evaluated.

MENSTRUAL HEALTH PROBLEMS IN SPECIAL POPULATIONS

In an effort to identify a population of women who might be at risk for the development of menstrual health problems, a group of 22 young women who had suffered a traumatic spinal cord injury of at least one year duration and had experienced a return of normal menstrual cycles were interviewed about their menstrual cycle function and hygiene practices (Reame, Note 5). Almost 70% of the subjects were injured at the cervical level producing some degree of quadriplegia. Twenty of the subjects were permanently confined to a wheel chair. Seven had indwelling catheters and 8 used intermittent catheterization. Urinary tract infections (40%) and muscle spasms (85.7%) were the major health problems and reasons for chronic use of medication such as sedatives, muscle relaxants and antibiotics.

Although 60% of the sample reported reduced vaginal sensation following injury, the majority of subjects (72%) chose to wear tampons as the primary menstrual hygiene product. There was no clear-cut favorite brand of tampon. Reasons for preference for tampons over pads included less chance of skin breakdown, odor, interference with catheterization, and leakage. Two women with limited hand dexterity cited greater ease of insertion with the O.B. digital tampon and the Kotex stick applicator.

When subjects were grouped according to level of injury, the mean duration of tampon wear was significantly longer for both high (9.5 hours) and low (9.0 hours) cervical lesion groups as compared to the noncervical lesion group (2.96 hours). This difference appeared related to the need for assistance with menstrual flow management. More than 90% of the women with cervical injuries required assistance with tampon insertion. In several instances, women reported that tampons were changed only with their morning care and at bedtime when help was available. Two women in this group reported the regular use of two super-absorbent tampons tied together and worn for up to 15 hours. Ten of the 16 tampon users (62%) wore tampons on an overnight basis.

In spite of the high incidence of chronic vaginal and urinary tract infections for the total group (41% having 3 or more per year), there was still a significant relationship demonstrated for tampon use. Tampon users who wore them on an overnight basis had a significantly greater incidence of urinary tract infections compared to those who switched to pads at night. Recommendations have been made by the CDC and FDA on how to use tampons to decrease the risk of developing toxic shock syndrome. These preventive measures include changing tampons every 4 to 6 hours and the use of pads on light days and at night (MMWR, 1980). In a study of tampon and pad usage among a multi-ethnic group of 186 able-bodied women in Hawaii, the mean frequency of tampon change was 4.5 hours (Ritz, McGee, & Coleman, Note 7). The pattern of tampon use in spinal cord injured women suggests that they may be less able to follow the recommendations of the CDC and more likely to be at risk for menstrual health problems because of longer or shorter than recommended length of tampon wear, overnight use, and reduced vaginal sensation.

It is clear from the above studies that menstrual health has emerged as an important clinical entity with far-reaching medical, social, political, and commercial implications. Future research should be directed to a better understanding of the physiology of menstruation, especially as it is effected by technological advances in the management of menstrual flow.

REFERENCE NOTES

1. Marlowe, D.E., Weigle, R.M., & Stauffenberg, R.S. *Measurement of tampon absorbancy—test method evaluation.* Food and Drug Administration, Bureau of Medical Devices, Report 81-013. May, 1981. Available from: Center for Medical Device Analysis, 8757 Georgia Ave., Silver Spring, Maryland 20910.

2. Reame, N.E. Factors affecting the composition of menstrual fluid. Paper presented to Kimberly-Clark Corp. Research and Development Staff, Neenah, Wisconsin, November 7, 1979.

3. Reame, N.E. Sex and menstrual function. Ninth Annual Conference on Psychosomatic Obstetrics and Gynecology, Philadelphia, March 25, 1981a.

4. Reame, N.E. Menstrual tampon absorbancy as viewed by scanning electron microscopy. Society for Menstrual Cycle Research Conference on Menarche. New Rochelle, New York, June 12, 1981b.

5. Reame, N.E. Menstrual cycle function and hygiene practices of women after traumatic spinal cord injury. Sixth Midwest Nursing Research Society Conference. Columbus, Ohio, April 9, 1982.

6. Reingold, A. Toxic Shock Syndrome Task Force, Bacterial Diseases Division Centers for Disease Control, Atlanta, Georgia. Personal communication.

7. Ritz, S.E., McGee, R.I., & Coleman, J.T. Patterns of tampon and pad usage in a select group of women in Hawaii. Paper presented at the American Public Health Association, Los Angeles, California, November 1, 1981.

REFERENCES

Andreev, D. Menstrual disturbances after interruption. *Folia Medica Cracoviensia* 1970, *12,* 263-265.

Barer, A.P, & Fowler, W.M. The blood loss during normal menstruation. *American Journal of Obstetrics and Gynecology,* 1936, *31,* 979-983.

Beller, F.K. Observations on the clotting of menstrual blood and clot formation. *American Journal of Obstetrics and Gynecology,* 1971, *111,* 535-546.

Beller, F.K., & Schweppe, K.W. Review on the biology of menstrual blood. In: F.K. Beller, & G.F.B. Schumacher (Eds.). *The biology of the fluids of the female genital tract,* New York: Elsevier North Holland, 1979.

Burnhill, M.S., & Birnberg, C.H. The contents of menstrual fluid. *American Journal of Obstetrics and Gynecology,* 1965, *92,* 183-88.

Bussing, H.J. Zur Biochemie des Menstrualblutes. *Zentralblatt fur Gynaekologie,* 1957, *79,* 456-560.

Champneys, F.H. *Painful menstruation.* London: H.K. Lewis, 1891.

Christiaens, G.C.M.L., Sixma, J.J, & Haspels, A. A. Fibrin and platelets in menstrual discharge before and after the insertion of intrauterine contraceptive device. *American Journal of Obstetrics and Gynecology,* 1981, *140,* 793-98.

Cohen, R. *National Consumer's League Bulletin,* March-April, 1982, Issue No. 131, 3.

Cole, S.K., Billewicz, W.Z., & Thomson, A.M. Sources of variation in menstrual blood loss. *Journal of Obstetrics and Gynaecology of the British Commonwealth,* 1971, *78,* 933-39.

Collins, R.K. Tampon-induced vaginal laceration. *Journal of Family Practice,* 1979, *9,* 127-128.

Consumer Reports. Menstrual tampons and pads. March 1978, *43,* 127-31.

Couture, M.L. Freund, M., & Sedlis, A. The normal exfoliative cytology of menstrual blood. *Acta Cytologica,* 1979, *23,* 85-89.

Davis, J.F., Chesney, J., Wand, P.J., & LaVenture, M. Toxic-shock syndrome. *New England Journal of Medicine,* 1980, *303,* 1429-35.

Ebert, C., Beller, F.K., Schweppe, K.W., & Wagner, H. Biochemistry of menstrual blood. In: F.K. Beller, & G.F.B. Schumacher (Eds.). *The biology of the fluids of the female genital tract.* New York: Elsevier North Holland, 1979.

Friedman, N. The truth about tampons. *New West,* 1980, *5,* 33-38.

Friedman, N. Everything you must know about tampons. New York: Berkely Books, 1981.

Friedrich, E.G., & Siegesmund, K.A. Tampon-associated vaginal ulcerations. *Obstetrics and Gynecology,* 1980, *55,* 149-56.

Friedrich, E.G. Tampon effects on vaginal health. *Clinical Obstetrics and Gynecology,* 1981, *24,* 395-406.

Frisch, R. Fatness, menarche, and fertility. In S. Golub (Ed.) *Menarche.* Lexington, Massachusetts: D.C. Heath, 1983.

Geist, S.H. The morphology of normal menstrual blood and its diagnostic value. *Surgery, Gynecology & Obstetrics,* 1929, *49,* 145-149.

Grimes, D.A. Estimating vaginal blood loss. *Journal of Reproductive Medicine,* 1979, *22,* 190-2.

Hallberg, L., & Nilsson, L. Constancy of individual menstrual blood loss. *Acta Obstetrica et Gynecologica Scandinavica,* 1964, *43,* 352-59.

Hallberg, L., Hogdahl, A.M., Nilsson, L., & Rybo, G. Menstrual blood loss: A population study. *Acta Obstetrica et Gynecologica Scandinavica,* 1966, *45,* 320-356.

Haynes, P.J., Hodgson, H., Anderson, A.B.M., & Turnbull, A.C. Measurement of menstrual blood loss in patients complaining of menorrhagia. *British Journal of Obstetrics and Gynecology,* 1977, *84,* 763-68.

Hefnawi, F. et al. The benefit of lactation amenorrhea as a contraceptive. *International Journal of Gynecology and Obstetrics.* 1977, *15,* 60-65.

Hinselmann, H. Der AusstoBungsmechanismus des menstrualblutes. *Zentralblatt fuer Gynaekologie,* 1925, *49,* 2386-2387.

Hytten, F.E., Cheyne, G.A., & Klopper, A.I. Iron loss at menstruation. *Journal of Obstetrics and Gynecology of The British Commonwealth.* 1964, *71,* 255-59.

Jeffcoate, N. *Principles of gynaecology,* 4th edition, London: Butterworths, 1975.

Macht, D.I. Further historical and experimental studies on menstrual toxin. *American Journal of Medical Science.* 1943, *206,* 281-305.

Morbidity and Mortality Weekly Report. Update on toxic shock. Sept 19, 1980, *29,* 441-45.

Moghissi, K.S., & Syner, F.N. The effect of seminal protease on sperm migration through the cervical mucus. *International Journal of Fertility.* 1970, *15,* 43-49.

Moghissi, K.S. The cervix in infertility. *Clinical Obstetrics and Gynecology.* 1979, *22,* 43-49.

Newton, J., Barnard, G., & Collines, W. A rapid method for measuring menstrual blood loss using automatic extraction. *Contraception.* 1977, *16,* 269-85.

Ober, K.G., Die Behandlung der unzulanglichen Keimdrusenfunktion. In: Seitz-Amreich II. S. 726 ff. Urban and Schwarzenberg, Berlin, 1952.

Pena, E.F. Menstrual protection: Advantages of the menstrual cup. *Obstetrics and Gynecology.* 1962, *19,* 684-86.

Pickles, V.R., Hall, W.J., Best, F.A., & Smith, G.N. Protaglandins in endometrium and menstrual fluid from normal and dysmenorrheic subjects. *British Journal of Obstetrics and Gynecology.* 1965, *72,* 185-92.

Poon. C.H., Moyer, D.L., Forineo, R.V. & Shaw, S.T. Studies on menstrual blood loss in intact and experimental rhesus monkeys. *Journal of Medical Primatology.* 1973, *2,* 353-63.

Preston, F.S., Bateman, S.C., Short, R.V., & Wilkinson, R.T. The effects of flying and of time changes on menstrual cycle length and on performance in airline stewardesses. In M. Ferin, F. Hallberg, R.M. Richart, & R.L. Vande Wiele (Eds.) *Biorhythms and human reproduction.* New York: Wiley, 1974.

Rybo, G. Clinical and experimental studies on menstrual blood loss. *Acta Obstetrica et Gynecologica Scandinavica,* supplement 7, 1966.

Schmidt, R.M. The effect of norethynodrel with mestranol on menstrual fluid volume. *Fertility and Sterility,* 1966, *17,* 381-385.

Schnatz, P.T. Bleeding and amenorrhea. In: S.L. Romney, M.J. Gray, A.B. Little et al., (Eds.) *Gynecology and obstetrics; The health care of women.* New York: McGraw-Hill, 1975.

Shands, K.N., Schmid, G.P., Dan, B.B., Blum, D., Guidotti, R.J., Hargrett, N.T., Anderson, R.L., Hill, D.L., Broome, C.E., Band, J.D., & Fraser, W.D. Toxic shock syndrome in menstruating women. *New England Journal of Medicine,* 1980, *303,* 1436-1442.

Shaw, S.T., Aaronson, D.E., & Moyer, D.L. Quantitation of menstrual blood loss-further evaluation of the alkaline hematin method. *Contraception.* 1972, *5,* 497-512.

Smith, O.W., & Smith, G.V. A fribrinolytic enzyme in menstruation and late pregnancy toxemia. *Science,* 1945, *102,* 253.

Stevenson, R.A., Culver, G.A., Stinson, J.C., & Kuenne, B.A. Quantity of menstrual flow. *Texas Reports on Biology and Medicine,* 1945, *3,* 371-381.

Stickel, M., & Zondek, B. Morphology and physical properties of menstrual blood. *Zeitschrift fuer Geburtshilfe und Gynakoologie,* 1920, *83,* 1-26

Sun, M. Use of "super-plus" tampons discouraged. *Science,* 1982, *216,* 1300.

Tatum, H.L. Metallic copper as an intrauterine contraceptive agent. *American Journal of Obstetrics and Gynecology,* 1973, *17,* 602-618.

Vander Vliet, W.L., & Hafez, E.S.E. Survival and aging of spermatozoa: A review. *American Journal of Obstetrics and Gynecology,* 1974, *118,* 1006-1015.

Zondek, B. Does menstrual blood contain a specific toxin? *American Journal of Obstetrics and Gynecology,* 1953, *65,* 1065-1068.

How Does Menstruation Affect Cognitive Competence and Psychophysiological Response?

Barbara Sommer, PhD

ABSTRACT. Studies of the effect of the menstrual cycle on standardized cognitive tasks, work and academic performance, perceptual-motor performance, and psychophysiological measures are reviewed. The weight of the evidence argues against a menstrual cycle effect on behavior. Studies of self report and of behaviors reflecting self confidence suggest that beliefs of menstrual debilitation remain in the population. Studies of atypical and deviant groups indicate a possible connection between behavior and the menstrual cycle.

Havoc produced by raging hormones is a joke to many. Yet, as a metaphor for the presumed effect of the menstrual cycle on female behavior, the raging hormone hypothesis lives. Brought to public attention in 1970 by a presidential candidate's physician (Barnes, 1971), raging hormones became the "female glandular system" in a Latin American diplomat's verbal attack on Prime Minister Thatcher concerning her response to the Argentine invasion of the Falklands (Isla Malvinas) in 1982. Concern about menstrual effects on behavior continues in legal circles with the premenstrual syndrome defense, of long use in France, and currently revived in Great Britain and the United States. The increasing employment of women outside the home has stimulated scientific research on the effects of menstruation. The old questions are disinterred with each cycle of concern for women's rights. Because the menstrual cycle is such a clear biologically distinguishing feature between the sexes, its correlates, concomitants, accompaniments, and ramifications, and implications have become intrinsically bound up with issues of gender equality.

CURRENT BELIEFS

We have become more open in our discussion of menstruation. The occurrence of the Toxic Shock Syndrome has done much to break down the secrecy and taboos surrounding menstruation; although at the same time has reinforced an ages-old myth of menstruation as dangerous. In 1981 the Tampax Corporation, a manufacturer of tampons, commissioned a study of attitudes toward menstruation and awareness of Toxic Shock Syndrome (The Tampax Report, 1981). The report is based on a survey of 1,034 Americans, a representative sample of the population over age 14. Interviews were done by telephone. Some of the items measured beliefs about the restrictions of menstruation. Selected questions and responses are shown in Table 1.

Survey results indicated that women are perceived as more emotional while menstruating, but not as less able to think, to work, or to engage in regular physical activities. However, a sizeable minority believe women cannot function normally while menstruating. Looking closely at Table 1, one sees that 35 percent believe menstruation affects a woman's ability to think and 26 percent believe women cannot function as well at work when menstruating.

Overall, there was a high level of agreement between the attitudes of men and women. However, one-third of the males surveyed disagreed with the statement that women can function as well at work while they're menstruating, compared with nineteen percent

Table 1

SELECTED ITEMS AND RESPONSE RATES FROM THE TAMPAX SURVEY, ITEM 11

	Agree Strongly	Tend to Agree	Tend to Disagree	Disagree Strongly
Women are more emotional when they are menstruating.	58	29	8	5
Women can function as well at work when they're menstruating.	48	26	17	9
Menstruation does not affect a woman's ability to think.	48	17	17	18
Women do not need to restrict their physical activities while menstruating.	44	26	20	10

of the females surveyed. While impairment is a minority view, these percentages represent a substantial number of individuals. If applied to the total U.S. population, they indicate that over 45 million Americans believe that women cannot function as well at work while menstruating, and over 60 million believe menstruation affects a woman's ability to think. It is important to point out that these figures represent a belief in impairment but not necessarily total debilitation. Respondents felt there was an effect, but the strength of the effect was not measured (see wording of the possible responses in Table 1).

While 87 percent agreed with the statement that women are more emotional while menstruating, when asked specifically about their last menstrual period (males were asked about wife/girlfriend's last period), 42 percent reported *no* mood changes or changes in personality during menstruation, and 58 percent said *no* such changes occurred during the week preceding menstruation.

The issue of whether or not menstrual cycle variables have a negative effect on women's thinking and on work behavior can be reduced to a series of factual questions:

—What is the evidence for impairment in thinking?
—What is the evidence for menstrual impairment in actual performance?
—What do laboratory studies reveal about the effect of menstruation on sensory and motor processes?
—Is there validity to the claims of increased psychopathology such as mental breakdown and criminal behavior around the time of menstruation?

There is a general bias in the research literature which favors the report of positive findings. Studies accepting the null hypothesis are treated with skepticism by editors. Most studies are designed to present and support specific hypotheses. Their rejection is often of little note. Otherwise, one could devise preposterous hypotheses, show that they are not confirmed, and publish the results. While in many areas it is reasonable to keep the literature clear of such studies, work on the menstrual cycle is of another sort. As the usual hypotheses tested are of some alteration, often of a decrement in performance, and have important implications for generalizations about women, publication of results failing to document change are of equal importance. Within the last ten years more studies have been published which report no phase effects. Yet, in doing this review I found a number of unpublished studies (some are listed in Table 3), most of them dissertations. Nearly all of them failed to document cyclic differences in performance. One wonders how many other studies rejecting the hypothesis of premenstrual and menstrual change have never reached print. It is possible that the reports of the cyclic fluctuation simply represent the one-in-twenty chance (using the .05 level of significance) of positive findings resulting from sampling error and other chance variation.

STANDARDIZED COGNITIVE TASKS AND PERCEPTUAL-MOTOR PERFORMANCE

There have been numerous studies of the effects of the menstrual cycle on standardized cognitive tasks and perceptual-motor function. Throughout this review, unless otherwise indicated, subjects of the studies reported are women who were not using oral contraceptives and who had regularly occurring menstrual cycles. The term *perimenstrual* is sometimes used to refer to the combined premenstrual and menstrual phases.

Table 2 lists the studies and shows the various measures used. In some studies a battery of tests was given and multiple measures were obtained from the same subject sample. Out of a total of sixteen published studies, most in journals using outside reviews, seven reported menstrual cycle phase effects. Two reported changes on some measures, but not on others; seven showed no differences in performance in relation to menstrual cycle phase.

Looking at the specific measures, of the 48 tests used, 35 showed no relationship between performance and the menstrual cycle. Of the thirteen measures fluctuating over the cycle, only three indicated perimenstrual impairment. Two of these are directly contradictory—Kopell, Lunde, Clayton, Moos and Hamburg (1969) found that time interval estimates were longer premenstrually, while Montgomery (1979) reported that shorter estimates of time intervals were produced premenstrually. Four other studies of time estimation reported no phase differences (Schwank, 1971; Zimmerman & Parle, 1973; Little & Zahn, 1974; Gamberale, Strindberg & Wahlberg, 1975). The Silverman and Zimmer (1975) finding of verbal disfluencies in the premenstrual phase remains with support from Komnenich (1974). However, contradictory evidence is provided by Golub (1976).

Four studies showed improved performance associated with the period around menstruation (Wuttke et al., 1973; Rodin, 1976; Munchel, 1979; Jones, Jones, & Hatcher, 1980). In two of these (Rodin, 1976; Jones et al., 1980) comparisons were between rather than within subjects. In the Rodin study, degree of menstrual symptomatology was varied and subjects were made anxious (threatened with mild electric shock). The menstrual enhancement only occurred in the treatment group. Subjects used as controls did not show any phase effects. Webster (1979) was unable to replicate Rodin's cognitive enhancement effect. Munchel also deliberately manipulated expectation. In the Jones et al. (1980) study the comparison groups (menstruating versus midcycle) differed in age and lacked additional controls for confounding factors. Thus, these studies do not provide a convincing data base for assuming a menstrual enhancement of performance. However, they are important because they illustrate the variability in results. They serve to underscore the generalization that perceptual-motor and cognitive performance as measured on standardized tests has little to do with the menstrual cycle, for, if in fact no relationship exists, one will occasionally find results in either direction by chance.

Some of the studies surveyed in Table 2 also included measures of reaction time (see Table 3). These are treated separately in the psychophysiological section of this review for two reasons. One is that several of the studies, particularly those on simple reaction time, have much in common with sensory threshold studies. Secondly, there are enough studies of reaction time so that the results have some comparability and may be considered replications.

Studies of higher level intellectual performance such as critical thinking and complex problem solving support the conclusion that intellectual function in normal healthy women is stable and independent of the fluctuation of the menstrual cycle (Lough, 1937; Wickham, 1958; Sommer, 1972a).

REAL WORLD STUDIES

Work Performance

Studies of the effect of menstruation on work performance are few. Redgrove (1971) studied the work output of eight women laundry workers over 25 complete cycles. She was able to make a detailed analysis for four of them and found no effects of menstrual

Table 2

RESULTS FOR STANDARDIZED COGNITIVE AND PERCEPTUAL-MOTOR TASKS

Studies showing menstrual cycle phase effects	Measures: Results
Kopell, et al., 1969	Time interval estimation: Longer intervals produced premenstrually
Montgomery, 1979	Time interval estimation: Shorter intervals produced premenstrually
Silverman & Zimmer, 1975	Verbal fluency (extemporaneous speech): Premenstrual increase in disfluencies
Kommenich, et al., 1978	Backward subtraction: Poorer performance in preovulatory phase
	Embedded Figures Test: Poorer performance in preovulatory phase
Klaiber, et al., 1974	Rod and Frame Test: Chance in response from preovulatory to post-ovulatory phase
Wuttke, et al., 1976	Simple arithmetic: Increased speed in luteal phase, optimum performance premenstrually
Dor-Shav, 1976	Human Figure Drawing: Better in postovulatory phase
	Embedded Figures Test: Better performance in postovulatory phase

Table 2 (continued)

Studies showing menstrual cycle phase effects	Measures: Results
Cormack and Sheldrake, 1974	Use of Objects Test: Preovulatory group scored higher than postovulatory group
	Verbal Task: Preovulatory group scored higher than postovulatory group
Jones, et al., 1980	Progressive Matrices: Menstruating group performed better than non-menstruating group
	Verbal Task: Menstruating group performed better than nonmenstruating group
Komnenich, 1974 (unpublished)	Verbal fluency (extemporaneous speech): Menstrual and postovulatory increase in disfluencies
Snyder, 1978 (unpublished)	Reflectivity/Impulsivity: Shorter response latency midcycle

Table 2 (continued)

Studies showing no phase differences in performance	Measures:	Results
Golub, 1976	Ability to reason	
	Fitting concepts to data	
	Rote memory	
	Ability to think rapidly of appropriate wording	
	Anagrams	
	Ideational fluency	
	Semantic elaboration	
	Ability to produce words from a restricted area of meaning	
	Semantic fluency and flexibility	
	Length estimation	
	Speed of closure	
	Flexibility of closure	

Table 2 (continued)

Studies showing no phase differences in performance	Measures:	Results
Gamberale, et al., 1975	Letter elimination	
	Perceptual speed	
	Stroop Color Word (without perceptual conflict)	
	Stroop Color Word (with perceptual conflict)	
	Time estimation	
Rodin, 1976	Digit symbol substitution	
	Stroop Color Word interference test	
	Anagrams	
	Unsolvable puzzles	
Zimmerman and Parlee, 1973	Digit Symbol (WISC)	
	Time estimation	
Komnenich, et al., 1978	Stroop Color Reading (noninterference)	
	Stroop Color Naming (noninterference)	
	Digit Symbol (WISC)	
Silverman and Zimmer, 1976	Verbal fluence (oral reading)	
Little and Zahn, 1974	Time estimation	

61

Table 2 (continued)

Studies showing no phase differences in performance	Measures:	Results
Wickham, 1958	Mechanical comprehension	
	Assembly of parts using diagram	
	Squares test (spatial task)	
	Spelling	
	Synonyms and rhymes	
	Arithmetic	
Sommer, 1972a	Watson-Glaser Critical Thinking	
Munchel, 1979 (unpublished)	Pursuit rotor with arithmetic	
	Concept formation	
	Unsolvable puzzle	
Altenhaus, 1978 (unpublished)	Subtraction	
	Solvable and unsolvable puzzles	
Sommer, 1972b (unpublished)	Speed of closure	
	Flexibility of closure	
	Addition	
	Visualization	

Table 2 (continued)

Studies showing no phase differences in performance	Measures:	Results
Snyder, 1978 (unpublished)	Flexibility of closure	
	Rod and Frame Test	
	Embedded Figures Test	
DiNardo, 1975 (unpublished)	Letter Series Test	
Schwank, 1971 (unpublished)	Time estimation	
Lederman, 1974 (unpublished)	Cognitive battery	
McKenna, 1974 (unpublished)	Perceptual-motor tasks	
Webster, 1979 (unpublished).	Cognitive tasks	

cycle phase on job performance. The same negative findings were obtained for nine punchcard operators and three typists, using a four-phase division of the menstrual cycle (dividing each individual's cycle into four phases of equal length).

Smith (1950a) studied the work performance of 38 women in aircraft, parachute, and garment factories during wartime production (World War II). He analyzed the independent ratings made by foremen. He used both a dichotomous analysis (menstrual vs. nonmenstrual) and a four-phase division of the cycle (5-day premenstrual phase, menstrual bleeding phase, 7-day postmenstrual phase and the remainder as intermenstrual phase). No phase differences were found in the ratings of work performance. In a second study he evaluated the quality and quantity of production, and again using both the dichotomous and four-phase divisions found little variation among 29 aircraft workers over a period of 41 days (Smith,1950b). While he found some incidence of lower production premenstrually on those tasks which possessed a high level of mental difficulty, this was counteracted by a higher level of work performance menstrually. Where significant differences did occur, they were more closely connected with situational variables than with menstrual ones.

Seward in her 1944 *Psychological Bulletin* review and 1946 book summarized the existing research on performance and the menstrual cycle and concluded that the studies to date demonstrated an absence of menstrual cycle effects on simple tasks and on choice reaction time and learning. The Smith study belongs with those in that it was probably motivated by concern about women's work in the wartime production effort. Little more was done until the resurgence of interest in women's work performance kindled by the women's movement of the late 1960s and 1970s, and fed by speculations of sociobiologists. In most subsequent studies the research settings have been the laboratory rather than the field as illustrated by the cognitive and psychomotor studies reviewed above.

Academic Performance

Dalton (1960) reported a decline in examination scores of schoolgirls, ages 11 to 17 years, in the premenstrual and menstrual phases (five days each). Although 27 percent of the students showed the drop, 17 percent improved their performance and 56 percent showed no change. As there was no statistical evaluation of these differences, the conclusion of perimenstrual impairment is an overstatement. In a second study Dalton (1968) examined the scores of students in England on advanced (A) and ordinary (O) level standardized examinations. The major flaw in this study was that on the A-level examinations she analyzed the grades assigned to 180 papers obtained from 34 individuals. This method puts a disproportionate weight on individuals submitting more papers. An average score per person for each phase should be calculated, and then the phase comparisons made. She reported that the average mark was three percent lower for those in the premenstrual and menstrual phases, that the pass rate was thirteen percent lower, and the distinction rate nine percent lower, compared with those in the intermenstrual phases. Given the confounding, those percentages are impossible to interpret. Also, it is important to note that these are not based on the same persons, that is, a between-group comparison is being made between those in one phase with those in another. The same type of confounding of more scores for some than for others occurred in the analysis of the O-level examinations where she compared scores on 162 papers from 91 individuals. In the same paper Dalton stated that the stress of exams (her inference) brought about an alteration in the cycle length in 42 percent of the young women. It appears that more of them than expected by chance were menstruating during the examination week. If test anxiety or some other factor brought about menstruation, it does not make sense to claim that being in the premenstrual or menstrual phase was the cause of the diminished performance, if in fact such a decrement did exist in the majority of the students studied—an assertion which is not supported by the data presented. Dalton herself stated that the alleged handicap was not evenly distributed among those studied.

Sommer (1972a) analyzed students' scores on biweekly psychology examinations which were assigned standardized scores. Each woman's cycle was divided into four phases of equal length. Comparisons were made both between groups (comparing the test performance of women in each cycle phase for each of three examinations) and within the group (comparisons of the individual's scores across her menstrual phases) for a total of 101 women. There was no relationship between performance and menstrual cycle phase. Students were not more likely to show their lowest scores in the premenstrual-menstrual phases compared with the two midcycle quarters.

Bernstein (1977) also studied performance on biweekly psychology examinations. Controlling for scholastic ability and motivation for 125 women, she found no difference in performance between tests taken in the perimenstrual phase (4 days prior to onset and the first 4 days of menstruation) and intermenstrual phase (all other days).

Walsh, Budtz-Olsen, Leader, and Cummins (1981) analyzed the examination scores of 244 female medical students and 97 paramedical students ranging in age from 17 to 27. Phase designations were menstrual (day 2 of menses), premenstrual (5 days before menses), luteal (15 days before menses) and midfollicular (midway between menstrual and luteal). Scores were examined for examinations which took place on or within one day of the above categories. For each person a difference score was computed for each of the four critical days listed above the average of other examinations taken. Thus, each subject served as her own control. No performance effects were found relative to cycle phase. In other words there was not a greater difference between the phase-designated scores and the average score at any particular time in the cycle. There was no relationship between performance and neuroticism as measured on the Eysenck Personality Inventory, nor a relationship between performance and menstrual symptomatology.

The weight of evidence on academic performance is clearly against an impairment model of menstruation.

Other Behaviors

Tuch (1975) reported that among 95 women who brought their children to a hospital pediatric outpatient department, 51 percent were in the premenstrual or menstrual phase of the cycle, defined as 5 days before and 6 days following menstruation. The expected percentage would be 39 percent. The difference was statistically reliable, although it is not clear why Tuch selected that particular phase designation, i.e., why five days prior and six days after menses? While both groups described their children as equally ill, examining physicians judged the children of the premenstrual and menstrual mothers as less ill. Sixty-one percent of the perimenstrual women brought in children who had been sick less than three days, while the corresponding percentage for the intermenstrual mothers was 35 percent.

Dalton (1966) surveyed mothers bringing their children to a general practitioner for treatment of minor coughs and colds. Using 4-day menstrual segments based on a 28-day cycle, 49 of the mothers (54%) were either in the premenstrual or menstrual phase. Chance expectancy for women to be in one or the other using 4-day designations is 29 percent.

The implication of these two studies is that judgments about illness, or perhaps worrying about one's child, is associated with menstruation. In this type of study it is difficult to disentangle the cognitive component (judgment) from affective ones.

Doty and Silverthorne (1975) found that women college students were more likely to volunteer to serve as subjects in a psychology experiment when in the ovulatory phase of the cycle than when in any of four other phases (menstrual, preovulatory, postovulatory, and premenstrual). Ovulatory phase was determined by subtracting fourteen days from subjects' self-reported cycle length and including the two days before and following estimated time of ovulation. Parlee (1975) contacted college women and asked them to participate in a psychological experiment. Of the 44 volunteers, more were in each of two midcycle phases than were in either the premenstrual or menstrual phases. While the results are similar to those of Doty and Silverthorne, the interpretation is limited by the fact that the menstrual status of twelve women who refused participation was not known. Also, nine who had volunteered had not menstruated in 28 days and were eliminated from the study. Some of them might have been premenstrual.

What the perception of illness in children and the volunteering studies have in common is that they may be measuring changes in self-confidence. The premenstrual and menstrual women may feel less competent or less able to evaluate their child's illness or to perform in a psychology experiment.

SELF-REPORT STUDIES

An instrument which is frequently used in menstrual cycle research is the Menstrual Distress Questionnaire (MDQ) developed by Moos (1977). The MDQ is a checklist consisting of 47 items which represent eight factor of symptom cluster, two of which are relevant to this review—Concentration and Behavior Change. The *Concentration* factor has eight specific symptoms: insomnia, forgetfulness, confusion, lowered judgment, difficulty concentrating, distractibility, accidents, and lowered motor coordination. The *Behavior Change* factor is represented by five items: lowered work performance; take naps, stay in bed; stay at home; avoid social activities; and decreased efficiency. The other six factors on the MDQ are Pain, Water Retention, Autonomic Reactions, Negative Affect, Arousal, and a Control cluster.

Ruble and Brooks-Gunn (1979) in their review of studies using the MDQ found a great deal of inconsistency in the results provided by this self-report measure. Overall, the studies do not show large average levels of menstrual and premenstrual changes compared with midcycle. Studies published subsequent to their review also support the generalization that the only consistent symptom clusters associated with the premenstrual and menstrual phases are Pain and Water Retention, and a trend toward premenstrual Negative Affect (Abplanalp, Donnelly, & Rose, 1979; Garling & Roberts, 1980; Most, Woods, Dery, & Most, 1981; Doty, Snyder, Huggins, & Lowry, 1981).

A recent study reporting evidence of debilitation is that of Kirstein, Rosenberg, & Smith (1980-81). They used the MDQ in a prospective study of 65 women over four months, and found a pattern of higher scores on the Concentration and Behavior Change factors around menstruation compared with midcycle. They also used another self-report measure, the Temporal Disorganization Scale (TDS), a 20-item measure of temporal indistinctness, impaired goal directedness, tracking dysfunction, desynchronization, and rate change durations. These scores were also higher premenstrually and menstrually. There are some problems with the study which limit its validity. The first is that while the study was prospective, it was not blind. Subjects were instructed to begin recording symptoms two weeks after the onset of their next menstruation. The forms were to be filled out weekly. The first page of the instruction booklet contained a calendar where the woman was to record the days she filled out the forms as well as to record onset and length of menstruation. The existence of negative expectations and attitudes towards menstruation is a possible source of bias in the responses. In an earlier review it was found that menstrual cycle effects on performance were more likely to be found when self-report was used in contrast with more objective assessment (Sommer, 1973). Also, in the Kirsten et al. study the phase designations varied in length. The premenstrual phase was designated as days -4 to -1 prior to menstruation; the other segments were -4 to -5 days prior to menstruation, menstrual duration, and postmenstrual duration. No basis for establishing these segments was given, for example, using a 5-day premenstrual designation, nor was it described as an *a priori* decision. Data were obtained from more women in some phases than in others; 65 in the two midcycle phases and 45 premenstrually and 49 menstrually. Given the length of the midcycle designation (one was nine days) and that the women were filling out symptom reports weekly and anonymously, it is possible that two reports might have come from the same respondent for the phase in question. Also, the study was done over a 4-month period. No mention was made of how scores were combined over the four months. The responses of the more diligent may be disproportionately reflected in the results. In addition to their between-group analyses with unequal sample sizes, a more accurate analysis would have been to perform a repeated-measures ANOVA for only those subjects for whom data were available from all four phases, and only one score (an average) per subject per phase should be used. This analysis was not done. According to the report, half of the sample responding in the premenstrual phase reported very little cognitive change.

Moos and Leiderman (1978) looked at symptom groupings among 579 women asked to describe their last menstrual cycle. Average age was 25.2 years. Nearly one-half (49) of the entire sample reported symptoms in only one of the eight factor areas of the MDQ. Of these 281 women, only two mentioned any symptoms connected with impaired concentration during menstruation, and another one during the premenstrual week. Seven reported symptoms from the Behavior Change factor menstrually, and another six premenstrually. The rarity of these complaints is shown by the contrast with 88 complaints of water retention menstrually and premenstrually. A second group (45 percent of the sample) reported symptoms on more than one of the 8-factor clusters. In these subgroups impairment of concentration was sometimes reported along with pain and negative affect. Behavior change was also associated in some cases with pain, both menstrually and premenstrually.

A logical hypothesis is that where cognitive impairment does occur, it is in conjunction with pain or negative affect. While severe pain is likely to impair concentration and bring about behavioral changes, the hypothesis of menstrual discomfort or dysphoria affecting concentration and mental performance has little support. Slade and Jenner (1980) in their study of choice reaction time selected for study women who complained of increased negative affect around the time of menstruation. They found only a slight hint of impairment on only the most difficult task. Hutt, Frank,

Mychalkiw, and Hughes (1980) failed to find phase differences in reaction time among four women suffering from premenstrual tension. Rodin (1976) found that a sample of women complaining of perimenstrual symptoms performed significantly better than a nonsymptom group on digit symbol and anagram tasks. Munchel (1979) selected a group of women who believed in performance decrements associated with menstruation; yet found that they did as well on concept formation and selected psychomotor tasks as did a group who did not believe that menstruation had a negative effect on performance. None of the studies reviewed have reported an association between objectively measured performance and reports of symptoms, and some studies have mentioned the absence of such an association (Ward, Stone, & Sandiman, 1978; Altenhaus, 1978). In other words even where the subject samples have included women who report menstrual distress or believe in the negative effects of menstruation the women tend not to show the expected decline in actual performance.

In summary it is not uncommon for women to report impaired concentration or behavior change in combination with other menstrual symptoms. However, these are reported with far less consistency than water retention and pain. There is a discrepancy between retrospective (after-the-fact) symptom reports and daily ratings made by the same persons. The retrospective reports are more likely to show the expected symptom fluctuation, that is, impairment or physical symptoms associated with menstruation; whereas daily reports often fail to show the cyclic variation (Sommer, 1972b; Friedmann, Katcher, & Brightman, 1978; Abplanalp, Donnelly, & Rose, 1979). Further, those women who do report symptoms in the premenstrual and/or menstrual phases do not show a pattern of impaired task performance at those times.

PSYCHOPHYSIOLOGICAL MEASURES

The studies reviewed thus far deal directly with the question of whether or not menstrual cycle variables affect cognitive function. Sensory and motor changes such as variations in threshold or in response rates as well as more central neural activities measured by EEG, are not generally defined as cognitive processes. However, they may provide information about cerebral events which might affect mental performance. The preceding statement is qualified because there is in fact no clear cognitive pattern associated with the menstrual cycle which needs to be explained. However, it is possible that those studies which do report cyclic effects are picking up behaviors connected with other neural activities. Many psychomotor tasks that researchers term "cognitive," because they appear to measure some aspect of mental ability, also measure visual processes and response rates. Thus, sensory-motor and sensory threshold studies are included here for completeness. Also reviewed are studies of spontaneous activity which probably say less about ability and more about motivation or subjective feelings of well-being and energy level. Like the sensory-motor variables, changes in activity might affect measured outcomes in performance. Not included are studies of physical endurance and athletic performance.

Reaction Time

Table 3 lists the studies and findings for both simple reaction time (response to a single signal) and choice reaction time (a choice among stimuli or responses must be made before responding). Twelve of the sixteen studies failed to show reliable phase effects. One of them (Schwank, 1971) claimed a trend toward a slower response rate in the premenstrual and menstrual phases. With the exception of Favreau (1973), those studies reporting phase effects involved choice reaction time, a more complex measure than simple reaction time, and those findings varied between premenstrual and menstrual slowing. The weight of the evidence is for no menstrual cycle effect on reaction time. In the few instances where phase effects did occur, they pointed toward a slowing of response speed around the time of menstruation.

Visual Sensitivity

Detection thresholds. In a study combining reaction time and visual sensitivity, Wuttke, Arnold, Becker, Creutzfeldt, Langenstein, and Tirsch (1976) measured speed of reaction when a constant light began to flicker. Among the sixteen respondents, response time was faster in the luteal phase when measured serum progesterone and estradiol were higher. They found a correlation between reaction time, as measured above, and increased levels of serum progesterone and estradiol. Subjects did not show faster

Table 3

SIMPLE AND CHOICE REACTION TIME STUDIES

Study	Number of Subjects	Results
Simple Reaction Time		
Pierson and Lockhart, 1963	25	No phase differences
Loucks and Thompson, 1968	44	No phase differences
Kopell, et al., 1969	8	No phase differences
Zimmerman and Parlee, 1973	14	No phase differences
Little and Zahn, 1974	12	No phase differences
Hunter, et al., 1979	18	No phase differences
Favreau, 1973 (unpublished)	6	Slower during menstruation
Choice Reaction Time		
Zimmerman and Parlee, 1973	14	No phase differences
Baisden and Gibson, 1975	17	No phase differences
Slade and Jenner, 1980	13	No phase differences
Hutt, et al., 1980		
Study I	12	No phase differences
Study II	4	No phase differences
Landauer, 1974	57	Slowest in premenstrual phase

Table 3 (continued)

Study	Number of Subjects	Results
Choice Reaction Time		
Gamberale, et al., 1975	12	Slower during menstruation
Hunter, et al., 1979	18	Slower in perimenstrual phase
Schwank, 1971 (unpublished)	10	No phase differences, but trend toward slower performance in perimenstrual phase

response rates in the preovulatory phase when estradiol alone was high.

Diamond, Diamond, and Mast (1972) studied the responses of four women in detecting a test light. They found peak sensitivity midcycle remaining high premenstrually, and dropping during menstruation. Ward et al., (1978) using a detection task where respondents reported the presence or absence of a dot found the best performance during the menstrual session and worst premenstrually, among 12 women. They also assessed mood and measured plasma estradiol, progesterone, luteinizing hormone and follicule-stimulating hormone. During the menstrual phase, when visual accuracy was highest, there was a correlation between estradiol level and the percentage of correct detection scores for the 12 subjects; estradiol accounted for 34 percent of the total variance of perceptual accuracy. However, on a pattern discrimination task (distinguishing between patterns of spaced dots and paired dots) there were no reliable differences associated with menstrual cycle phase, with a trend for better performance premenstrually. There was no relationship between the mood and performance measures.

Barris, Dawson, and Theiss (1980) evaluated scotopic threshold (responses of the rods) for five respondents across the midcycle shift in basal body temperature, analyzing data from three days prior to the temperature rise, using seven days in all. Scotopic visual sensitivity (night vision) increased only on the day of the temperature rise.

Two-flash fusion threshold. The two-flash fusion threshold is the point at which the observer reports two successive light flashes as one. It measures the capacity to make fine temporal discriminations, that is, to distinguish the two flashes even though they are occurring very close in time. A higher threshold reflects a failure to distinguish the two flashes until more time elapses between them. Threshold levels involve sensitivity to the stimuli as well as a number of other factors such as expectation, willingness to respond, and the influence of instructions. Thus a threshold determination is not always an accurate indication of sensory acuity.

Kopell et al. (1969) studying two-flash fusion in eight women found no reliable phase effects, but a trend toward decreased sensitivity premenstrually, although the greater sensitivity (point at which two flashes are seen as distinct) occurred in the preovulatory rather than postovulatory half of the cycle. Also working with paired flashes, DeMarchi and Tong (1972) found decreased sensitivity in the premenstrual phase, with an increase during menstruation and greatest sensitivity midcycle (N = 20). These results were confounded with a practice effect and in a replication Wong and Tong (1974) found no phase differences among eight subjects. Clare, Tong, Lyon, and Leigh (1976) found no difference comparing midcycle (day 14) with premenstrual phase (day 27) for eight subjects who also were given either a small dose of ethanol or a placebo drink. Braier and Asso (1980) using between-subjects design—one group was tested around menstruation (within four days of onset) and the other midcycle (mid third)—found a higher threshold in the perimenstrual group.

In three of the studies listed in Table 4 (Diamond et al., 1972; Wong & Tong, 1974; Wuttke et al., 1976) subjects using oral contraceptives were also tested, and in all three cases showed no fluctuation in response over the menstrual cycle.

The data on visual sensitivity tend towards supporting midcycle increases in sensitivity but vary among preovulatory and postovulatory segments. The patterns of response found within as well as between studies remain contradictory, e.g., Ward et al. (1978) in their well-designed study found different response patterns associated with different tasks—signal detection versus pattern discrimination. Either cyclic patterns are task specific, or extraneous variables contribute artifacts which are mixed in with small reliable differences. In any case the reliable patterns remain to be distinguished. Adding in data from other sensory studies does little to improve the clarity of the picture.

Auditory Sensitivity

Schubert, Meyer, and Washer (1975) measured auditory threshold in seven subjects in the menstrual (within 48 hours of onset), postmenstrual (days 7-9), and midcycle (days 14-16) phases. There were no threshold differences across phase. Haggard and Gaston (1978) measured sensitivity to a variety of auditory stimuli in twelve subjects—tone modulation (beats), octave mathing, frequency JND, and click lateralization. They used four phases covering the entire menstrual cycle. While a variety of fluctuations were found across subjects and tasks, no clear menstrual cycle phase relationship emerged.

Cox (1980) tested the hypothesis of a *decrease* in aural sensitivity associated with higher estrogen levels. Instead, he found lower sen-

Table 4

PSYCHOPHYSIOLOGICAL MEASURES

Measure

   Results   Study

Detection threshold

   Lower during menstrual phase; higher in premenstrual phase   Ward, et al., 1978

   Lower in preovulatory phase   Haggard and Gaston, 1978

   Lower midcycle and in premenstrual phase   Diamond, et al., 1972

   Lowest scotopic threshold (night vision) on day of basal body
      temperature rise   Barris, et al., 1980

Two-flash fusion threshold

   Lower in perimenstrual phase   Braier and Asso, 1980

   Lowest in premenstrual phase   DeMarchi and Tong, 1972

   Lowest in premenstrual phase   Kopell, et al., 1969

   No phase difference   Wong and Tong, 1974

   No phase difference   Clare, et al., 1976

Auditory threshold

   Higher during menstruation   Cox, 1980

   No phase difference   Haggard & Gaston, 1978

   No phase difference   Schubert, et al., 1975

Table 4 (continued)

Measure	
Results	Study

Olfactory threshold

Lower midcycle	Doty, et al., 1981
Lower midcycle	Mair, et al., 1978
Lower midcycle and in premenstrual phase	Vierling and Rock, 1967
No phase difference	Amoore, et al., 1975

GSR (Galvanic Skin Response)

Greater in preovulatory phase	Friedman and Meares, 1979
Greater in preovulatory phase (trend only)	Uno, 1973
Lower in postovulatory phase	Little and Zahn, 1974
No phase differences	Slade and Jenner, 1979
No phase differences	Zimmerman and Parlee, 1973

EEG (Alpha frequency)

Postovulatory increase	Creutzfeldt, et al., 1976
Postovulatory increase	Vogel, et al., 1971
Premenstrual decrease	Sugerman, 1970
Premenstrual increase	Leary and Batho, 1979

sitivity during menstruation, an effect attributed to increased fluid retention affecting the eustachian tube.

Olfactory Sensitivity

Vierling and Rock (1967) found two peaks of olfactory sensitivity to exaltolide, a musk-like odor, in 73 respondents—one peak around the expected time of ovulation and the other in the luteal phase approximately eight days prior to menses. However, Amoore, Popplewell, and Whissell-Buechy (1975) found no menstrual cycle variation. Mair, Bouffard, Engen, and Morton (1978) reported a midcycle increase in olfactory sensitivity to three of four odors measured over the entire cycle in twelve subjects.

Doty, Snyder, Huggins, and Lowry (1981) found support for increased sensitivity midcycle. There was a substantial positive correlation between serum estrogen levels and olfactory sensitivity for seventeen women studied every two days over two menstrual cycles. The surprise in their results was the occurrence of cyclic changes in olfaction among a comparison sample of six women using oral contraceptives; a finding which raises questions about the ovarian basis of sensory changes in olfaction.

Galvanic Skin Response (GSR)

The GSR measures skin resistance which is used as an indicator of neural arousal or responsiveness. Two electrodes are attached to the palm of the hand. They measure minute changes in perspiration on the skin. The procedure used in the following studies was to sound a tone and then measure change in GSR, generally expressed as skin conductance. One can measure the amplitude of the response itself, or habituation—when a previous response ceases to occur on presentation of the tone. The inference is made that responding with greater amplitude or requiring more trials to habituation reflects greater arousal or autonomic nervous system activation.

Zimmerman and Parlee (1973) found no phase differences among fourteen women studied across four phases: menstrual (days 1-4), follicular (days 6-12), luteal (days 17-21), and premenstrual (days 23-27). Little and Zahn (1974) divided the cycle into 10 segments and used a three-fold comparison: Low hormonal activity (deciles 1 and 2), ovulatory, maximum estrogen (deciles 4 and 5) and luteal, high progesterone (deciles 7, 8, and 9). GSR amplitude dropped significantly in the luteal phase in their sample of twelve women.

Uno (1973) using a between-subjects design tested thirty women in three groups: postmenses (days 5-7), preovulation (days 12-14), and premenses (days 24-26). There were no phase differences in skin conductance, but the amplitude of the response was greater in the postmenses (follicular) group than in the premenses group. Because of the wide range of individual differences, between-group measures should be viewed with caution. When sample size is small, a mean difference may reflect individual differences in overall responsiveness rather than phase differences. A number of researchers have commented on substantial individual differences in performance of psychophysiological and psychomotor tasks.

Slade and Jenner (1979) measured skin conductance in response to specific tasks in addition to the presentation of tones. After a period of rest, the fourteen subjects were required to move a ring along a complicatedly shaped wire (without touching the wire) for 2½ minutes during the presentation of white noise. After a rest period, they simultaneously solved arithmetic problems and did a 4-choice card sorting task for another 2½ minutes. Then, following a rest period, tones were sounded at random intervals. Difference scores were calculated between skin conductance during the tasks or tones, and the preceding rest periods. They used a four-fold cycle designation: menstrual (days 1-4), preovulatory (3-6 days before basal body temperature rise), postovulatory (1-6 days after rise in temperature), and premenstrual (5-1 days preceding onset of flow). While large differences between rest and activity levels were found, no phase effects occurred. It is of note that these fourteen subjects were selected for study because they specifically reported unpleasant premenstrual and menstrual symptoms.

Using a six-segment cycle division, Friedman and Meares (1979) studied habituation of GSR for 21 women over two menstrual cycles at one-week intervals. They also measured urinary estrogens and pregandiol. The level for the first three segments of the cycle (preovulatory) was high, i.e., more tones were presented before the GSR response stopped occurring, whereas in the latter three segments (postovulatory phase) habituation occurred more rapidly. From these results, they concluded that CNS arousal was higher in the preovulatory phase relative to the postovulatory phase. The shift was not observed in seven women who were using oral contraceptives. Their habituation pattern resembled that of the ovulating women in the last half of the cycle.

In summary, the GSR data are not entirely consistent. Where change is reported it indicates greater responsiveness, perhaps sensitivity, in the preovulatory compared with postovulatory segments of the cycle. There are no indications of changes associated only with the premenstrual-menstrual segments. As with the data on vision and olfaction, variations in response seem to have a more immediate connection with ovulation. However, when looking more closely at midcycle and measuring hormonal change either with basal body temperature change or urinary or serum assay, the findings are inconsistent.

Electroencephalogram (EEG) Changes

Studies of EEG patterns over the menstrual cycle yield inconclusive results (see Table 4). All used a within-subjects design where the same women were tested at different cycle phases.

Becker, Schwibbe, and Wuttke (1981) pursuing EEG and other changes reported by Creutzfeldt et al. (1976) and Wuttke et al. (1976) made further studies which suggest that small changes in psychophysiological responses and simple psychomotor performance may be connected with changes in body temperature rather than specific gonadal hormones. Progesterone increases body temperature. However, they found similar changes in performance in males injected with a pyrogenic substance. However, while Stenn and Klinge (1972) found a low, but reliable, correlation between arm movement and body temperature for women, the relationship did not hold for their small sample of three men.

Other Related Studies

A variety of studies aimed at finding changes in sensory sensitivity or CNS arousal have been done (Table 5). In many cases there have been no replications of findings. In other instances where there has been replication as with EEG, the findings differ. In some cases the researchers are simply using the menstrual cycle as a vehicle for testing hypotheses about neural functioning. They are not interested in the menstrual cycle per se, but instead study selected phases thereby limiting generalization over the entire cycle, for example, the studies of adrenergic function (Klaiber, Broverman, Vogel, Kobayashi, & Moriarty, 1971) and stimulus modulation (Baker, Kostin, Mishara, & Parker, 1979). Some researchers have attempt-

Table 5

OTHER MEASURES

Measure: Results	Study
Adrenocortical response to psychological stress: Greater responsiveness premenstrually	Marinari, et al., 1976
Acquisition of conditioned response measured by heartrate: Premenstrual group conditioned more readily	Vila and Beech, 1978
Shock aversion: Greatest sensitivity in preovulatory phase; lowest around ovulation	Tedford, et al., 1977
CNS arousal and responsiveness: Premenstrual increase	Wineman, 1971
Kinesthetic aftereffect: Increase at beginning and end of cycle	Baker, et al., 1979
Aneiseikonic body perception: Less distortion through lens as approach menstruation	Fisher, et al., 1969
Corneal sensitivity to touch: Less sensitivity premenstrually	Millodot & Lamont, 1974
Ratings of pleasantness of sugar solutions: Slightly higher ratings in postovulatory phase	Wright and Crow, 1972
Arm-hand steadiness: Greater midcycle	Zimmerman and Parlee, 1973

ed to establish hypotheses and organize discrepant findings under the rubric of changes in arousal or in activation-inhibition terms (Asso, 1978; Broverman, Vogel, Klaiber, Majcher, Shea, & Paul, 1981). However, the contradictory findings mitigate against the success of these attempts.

Spontaneous Motor Activity

Stenn and Klinge (1972) had subjects wear wristwatch-style actometers which measured arm movements (worn on the nonfavored hand) during day and night. Subjects were seven women over seventeen menstrual cycles. Using a 4-phase division of the cycle, they did not find significant cycle effects. They were not able to detect any cyclic pattern in activity, although none of the women showed an activity peak during the five days of menstruation, and both day and night arm movement peaks were more likely to occur during the second half of the cycle. They found a statistically reliable, but low, correlation (r = .217 for daytime and r = .216 for nighttime), between arm movement and basal body temperature (used as indicator of hormonal fluctuation).

Morris and Urdry (1970) studied 24 women who wore pedometers daily through three menstrual cycles, and nine others who participated for shorter periods of time. They reported a significant increase in activity midcycle with two lesser peaks menstrually and premenstrually (days 27 and day 2 following onset of flow). The pattern emerged only when the data for all women were combined. There was a great deal of variability both between subjects and within subjects across cycles.

Comment

It is very difficult to make clear generalizations about the psychophysiological data. Some studies report cyclic variations and others do not. Where variation is found, it tends to point to increased sensitivity or responsiveness midcycle and a reduction around the time of menstruation. However, the variations among findings are such that once could select studies to support almost any hypothesis one chose—sensitivity changes correlated with estrogens or progesterone, or both, or neither; increased sensitivity or arousal around menses or decreased sensitivity around menses, or no difference. In trying to make sense of the welter of data, some general problem areas emerge which must be dealt with if more clear findings are to emerge in future work.

One problem area is that of research agenda. Much of the research on psychophysiological as well as psychomotor variables was stimulated by a concern with explaining phenomena that were not consistent in the first place—the occurrence of behavioral and emotional disturbance in the premenstrual and/or menstrual phases. As evidenced in the introductory sections of many of the papers reviewed, disturbance or debilitation was assumed. The research was designed to investigate the causes of such disturbance. It may well be that the absence of consistent findings reflects the absence of consistent problems in the population under study.

There also is the issue of differing research agendas, and it may be misleading to make generalizations about the menstrual cycle as a whole and its effects on behavior from studies which are primarily concerned with other factors. There are two general groups of researchers who have published studies concerning the menstrual cycle. One group is comprised of those who are interested in the menstrual cycle itself in its entirety—physiology of the cycle, or the sociocultural and personal meanings associated with menstrual bleeding.

A second group consists of researchers interested in more broad areas of hormones and behavior, or in social psychology or anthropology, who see the menstrual cycle as an appropriate phenomenon for testing specific hypotheses. For the hormones and behavior area, the menstrual cycle is a convenient source of study as a naturally occurring incidence of hormonal fluctuation. An example of this approach is the study of Broverman, Vogel, Klaiber, Majcher, Shea and Paul (1981) on shifts in performance of simple highly-practiced tasks like color naming relative to performance of perceptual-restructuring tasks such as finding embedded figures. Social psychologists have used responses to menstruation to test hypotheses about attribution theory (Rodin, 1976; Ruble and Brooks-Gunn, 1979). Studying the menstrual cycle per se or looking at particular aspects of it as part of larger theoretical issues leads to differences in research design and findings which may not be comparable. Contradictory results may reflect the different questions being addressed. Researchers in the first group may be interested in testing hypotheses about menstrual impairment or the effects of the cycle on mood. In these cases the menstrual cycle or menstruation itself is the independent or predictor variable. The second group may use menstruation or symptoms associated with it as a dependent variable, as an outcome of changes in hormones, or a reflection of beliefs about menstruation. For example, Rubel (1977) reported that women convinced that they were about to menstruate reported symptoms of water retention and pain even when in fact they were not premenstrual. While this study demonstrates symptom perception in the absence of physiological change, and in the presence of psychological suggestion, it does not demonstrate that women experiencing water retention and pain are doing so only for psychological reasons. It does not disconfirm the hypothesis that metabolic changes lead to water retention. It simply provides another basis for the symptom reports. Pain and water retention are the factors which are most consistently reported in the premenstrual and menstrual phases on the MDQ. While Ruble's study tells us something about women's perception of menstrual events, it does not tell us anything about the effects of the menstrual cycle on behavior. Many of the studies involving the menstrual cycle do not deal directly with it as a variable influencing women's behavior. Clear statements of the purpose of research as well as the particular hypotheses being tested will make agendas more clear and allow a better grouping of findings and their implications.

A far more serious problem is the absence of replication. Few studies are replicated prior to publication, and after publication there is little motivation for either the originators or their colleagues to repeat the work. This lack leads to the inclusion of spurious findings in the literature. It is clear, given the body of research done thus far, that menstrual cycle effects are probably small, perhaps even ephemeral. If such effects are to be documented, replication is necessary to distinguish them from artifacts and spurious associations. At the present time it would be futile to attempt to spin a web of theory around the existing discrepant findings when so few have been exposed to the test of replication.

A third area of difficulty is the wide variation in phase designations. In doing the current review I have found much improvement in the specification of phases, but selection remains as heterogeneous as it was ten years ago (Sommer, 1973). This heterogeneity makes comparisons and conclusions across studies very difficult. An extremely useful contribution of the Society for Menstrual Cycle Research would be to establish recommended guidelines in the area of phase designation. Researchers would, of course, be free to use whatever phases they wished, but if in addition they would present results in accordance with generally accepted guidelines, a substantial improvement in the field would be made. Guidelines could be of two sorts—broad designations such as quarters or thirds, and more narrow ones such as 2-day intervals or tenths. Leaving the designation to *post hoc* determination opens up the possibility of spurious findings, that is, making the phase fit the results so as to support proposed hypotheses.

REAL LIFE PATHOLOGY

Friedman, Hurt, Arnoff and Clarkin (1980) reviewed studies drawing samples from populations which are defined as atypical, for example, the psychiatrically disabled, women who are involved in accidents and in crimes, attempted suicides, depressives, etc. They concluded that "within the universe of potential pathological-act committers, the paramenstrual period is a time of relatively high expectancy for the occurrence of the act in question" (page 733).

While there are studies which support this conclusion (d'Orban & Dalton, 1980; Glass, Heninger, Lansky, & Talen, 1971; Dalton, 1960), some of them were used to support a similar conclusion about women in general. This is increasingly rare because of the substantial amount of contradictory evidence generated over the last ten years. A series of well-designed studies of deviant groups, such as the mentally disturbed and persons with poor impulse control, remains to be done. Also, the scientific study of menstruation may influence processes accounting for links between menstruation and misbehavior. There may be an analogy with the demise of hysteria. Hysteria tends to be no longer real in the eyes of the lay public, and while cases do occur, they are not nearly as common as they were in the past. In part this may be due to differential diagnoses, but it also may be due to a more sophisticated public well-versed in the Freudian mysteries of the unconscious. Such may be the future of reports of menstrual impairment. As an increasing amount of public attention is paid, we may see an increase in the plea of sick behavior being caused by premenstrual tension, but a decline of menstrual debility in the population as people become more aware of scientific findings which argue against premenstrual and menstrual debilitation in most women.

CONCLUSION

Taking all of the reviewed studies in their entirety, the conclusion is that among the general population of women, menstrual cycle variables do not interfere with cognitive abilities—abilities of thinking, problem-solving, learning and memory, making judgments, and other related mental activities. There are indications that the hormonal fluctuations of the cycle are evidenced in small changes in sensory acuity and sensitivity, and that there may be small effects on motor activity. The data on these sensory-motor effects are neither clear nor consistent. The inconsistencies may be the result of the failure to replicate studies before they reach print. They may also stem from inconsistent phase designations and differences in the variables under study, for example, correlating behavior with measured hormone levels, or using basal body temperature to infer ovulation and then assuming a predictable pattern of hormone secretion, or simply assuming midcycle ovulation and its attendant hormonal changes. If further research is felt to be needed, those doing it should address these problems directly.

REFERENCES

Abplanalp, J. M., Donnelly, A. F., & Rose, R. M. Psychoendocrinology of the menstrual cycle: I. Enjoyment of daily activities and moods. *Psychosomatic Medicine,* 1979, *41,* 587-604.

Altenhaus, A. L. The effect of expectancy for change on performance during the menstrual cycle. *Dissertation Abstracts International,* 1978, *39*(2-B), 968.

Amoore, J. E., Popplewell, J. R., & Whissell-Buechy, D. Sensitivity of women to musk odor: No menstrual variation. *Journal of Chemical Ecology,* 1975, *1,* 291-297.

Asso, D. Levels of arousal in the premenstrual phase. *British Journal of Social and Clinical Psychology,* 1978, *17,* 47-55.

Baker, A. H., Kostin, I. W., Mishara, B. L., & Parker, L. Menstrual cycle affects kinesthetic aftereffect, an index of personality and perceptual style. *Journal of Personality and Social Psychology,* 1979, *37,* 234-246.

Baisden, A. G., & Gibson, R. S. Effects of the menstrual cycle on the performance of complex perceptual-psychomotor tasks. *Human Factors Society, 19th Proceedings,* 1975, 415-417.

Barnes, A. C. The opening of the second front: Dr. Berman and the ladies. *Obstetrics & Gynecology,* 1971, *37,* 320-322.

Barris, M. D., Dawson, W. W., & Theiss, C. L. The visual sensitivity of women during the menstrual cycle. *Documents in Opthalmology,* 1980, *49,* 293-301.

Becker, D., Schwibbe, M., & Wuttke, W. Effects of gonadal steroids on EEG and performance in the human. *Experimental Brain Research,* 1981, *Supp. 3,* 309-317.

Bernstein, B. E. Effect of menstruation on academic performance among college women. *Archives of Sexual Behavior,* 1977, *6,* 289-296.

Braier, J. R. & Asso, D. Two-flash fusion as a measure of changes in cortical activation with the menstrual cycle. *Biological Psychology,* 1980, *11,* 153-156.

Broverman, D. M., Vogel, W., Klaiber, E. L., Majcher, D., Shea, D., & Paul, V. Changes in cognitive task performance across the menstrual cycle. *Journal of Comparative and Physiological Psychology*, 1981, *95*, 646-654.

Clare, G., Tong, J. E., Lyon, R. G., & Leigh, G. Menstrual cycle and ethanold effects on temporal discrimination. *Perceptual & Motor Skills*, 1976, *42*, 1085-1086.

Cormack, M. & Sheldrake, P. Menstrual cycle variations in cognitive ability: A preliminary report. *International Journal of Chronobiology*, 1974, *2*, 53-55.

Cox, J. R. Hormonal influence on auditory function. *Ear & Hearing*, 1980, *1*, 219-222.

Creutzfeldt, O. D., Arnold, P. M., Becker, D., Langenstein, S., Tirsch, W., Wilhelm, H., & Wuttke, W. EEG changes during spontaneous and controlled menstrual cycles and their correlation with psychological performance. *Electroencephalography in Clincal Neurophysiology*, 1976, *40*, 113-131.

Dalton, K. Effect of menstruation on schoolgirls' weekly work. *British Medical Journal*, 1960a, *1*, 326-328.

Dalton, K. Menstruation and accidents. *British Medical Journal*, 1960b, *2*, 1425-1426.

Dalton, K. The influence of mother's menstruation on her child. *Proceedings of the Royal Society of Medicine*, 1966, *59*, 1014-1016.

Dalton, K. Menstruation and examinations. *Lancet*, 1968, *2*, 1386-1388.

DeMarchi, G. W. & Tong, J. E. Menstrual, diurnal, and activation effects on the resolution of temporally paired flashes. *Psychophysiology*, 1972, *9*, 362-367.

Diamond, M. Diamond, A., & Mast, M. Visual sensitivity and sexual arousal levels during the menstrual cycle. *Journal of Nervous and Mental Diseases*, 1972, *155*, 170-176.

DiNardo, P. G. Psychological correlates of the menstrual cycle. *Dissertation Abstracts International*, 1975, *36*(6-B), 3031.

d'Orban, P. T. & Dalton, J. Violent crime and the menstrual cycle. *Psychological Medicine*, 1980, *10*, 353-359.

Dor-Shav, N. K. In search of pre-menstrual tension: Note on sex-differences in psychological differentiations as a function of cyclical physiological changes. *Perceptual & Motor Skills*, 1976, *42*(3), 1139-1142.

Doty, R. L. & Silverthorne, C. Influence of menstrual cycle on volunteering behavior. *Nature*, 1975, *254*(5496), 139-140.

Doty, R. L., Snyder, P. J., Huggins, G. R., & Lowry, L. D. Endocrine, cardiovascular, and psychological correlates of olfactory sensitivity changes during the human menstrual cycle. *Journal of Comparative and Physiological Psychology*, 1981, *95*, 45-60.

Favreau, O. E. Menstrual cycles and sex differences. Paper presented at the *Annual Meeting of the Canadian Psychological Association*, 1973. Dept. de Psychologie, Université de Montreal, Montreal, Quebec, Canada.

Fisher, S. et al. Selective effects of the menstrual experience upon aniseikonic body perception. *Psychosomatic Medicine*, 1969, *21*, 365-371.

Friedman, J. & Meares, R. A. The menstrual cycle and habituation. *Psychosomatic Medicine*, 1979, *41*, 369-381.

Friedman, R. C., Hurt, S. W., Arnoff, M. S., & Clarkin, J. F. Behavior and the menstrual cycle. *Signs: Journal of Women in Culture and Society*, 1980, *5*, 719-738.

Friedmann, E., Katcher, A. H., & Brightman, V. J. A prospective study of the distribution of illness within the menstrual cycle. *Motivation and Emotion*, 1978, *2*, 355-367.

Gamberale, F., Strindberg, L., & Walhlberg, I. Female work capacity during the menstrual cycle: Physiological and psychological reactions. *Scandinavian Journal of Work and Environmental Health*, 1975, *1*, 120-127.

Garling, J. & Roberts, S. J. An investigation of cyclic distress among staff nurses. In A. J. Dan, E. A. Graham, & C. P. Beecher (Eds.), *The menstrual cycle: Volume I, A synthesis of interdisciplinary research*. New York: Springer Publishing, 1980, 305-311.

Glass, G. W., Heninger, G. R., Lansky, M., & Talen, K. Psychiatric emergency related to the menstrual cycle. *American Journal of Psychiatry*, 1971, *128*, 705-711.

Golub, S. The effect of premenstrual anxiety and depression on cognitive function. *Jounal of Personality and Social Psychology*, 1976, *34*, 99-104.

Haggard, M. & Gaston, J. B. Changes in auditory perception in the menstrual cycle. *British Journal of Audiology,* 1978, *12,* 105-118.

Hunter, S., Schraer, R., Landers, D. M., Buskirk, E. R., & Harris, D. V The effects of total oestrogen concentration and menstrual-cycle phase on reaction time performance. *Ergonomics,* 1979, *22,* 263-268.

Hutt, S. J., Frank, G., Mychalkiw, W., & Hughes, M. Perceptual-motor performance during the menstrual cycle. *Hormones and Behavior,* 1980, *14,* 116-125.

Jones, B. M., Jones, M. K., & Hatcher, E. M. Cognitive deficits in women alcoholics as a function of gynecological status. *Journal of Studies of Alcohol,* 1980, *41,* 140-146.

Kirstein, L., Rosenberg, G., & Smith, H. Cognitive changes during the menstrual cycle. *International Journal of Psychiatry in Medicine,* 1980-81, *10,* 339-346.

Klaiber, E. L., Broverman, D. M., Vogel, W., Kobayashi, Y., & Moriarty, D. Effects of estrogen therapy on plasma MAO activity and EEG driving responses of depressed women. *American Journal of Psychiatry,* 1972, *128,* 1492-1498.

Komnenich, P. Hormonal influences on verbal behavior in women. *Dissertation Abstracts International,* 1974, *35,* 3065B.

Komnenich, P., Lane, D. M., Dickey, R. P., & Stone, S. C. Gonadal hormones and cognitive performance. *Physiological Psychology,* 1978, *6,* 115-120.

Kopell, B., Lunde, D., Clayton, R., Moos, R., & Hamburg, D. Variations in some measures of arousal during the menstrual cycle. *Journal of Nervous and Mental Diseases,* 1969, *148,* 180-187.

Landauer, A.A. Choice decision time and the menstrual cycle. *Practitioner,* 1974, *213,* 703-706.

Leary, P. M. & Batho, K. Changes in electro-encephalogram related to the menstrual cycle. *South African Medical Journal,* 1979, *55,* 666,668.

Lederman, M. Menstrual cycle and fluctuation in cognitive-perceptual performance. *Dissertation Abstracts International,* 1974, *35,* 1388B-1389B.

Little, B. C. & Zahn, T. P. Changes in mood and autonomic functioning during the menstrual cycle. *Psychophysiology,* 1974, *11,* 579-590.

Loucks, J. & Thompson, H. Effect of menstruation on reaction time. *Research Quarterly,* 1968, *39,* 407-408.

Lough, E. M. A psychological study of functional periodicity. *Journal of Comparative Psychology,* 1937, *24,* 359-368.

Mair, R. G., Bouffard, J. A., Engen, T., & Morton, T. H. Olfactory sensitivity during the menstrual cycle. *Sensory Processes,* 1978, *2,* 90-98.

Marinari, K. T., Leshner, A. I., & Doyle, M. P. Menstrual cycle status and adrenocortical reactivity to psychological stress. *Psychoneuroendocrinology,* 1976, *2,* 213-218.

McKenna, W. B. The menstrual cycle, motivation, and performance. *Dissertation Abstracts International,* 1974, *64,* 1391B.

Millodot, M. & Lamont, A. Influence of menstruation on corneal sensitivity. *British Journal of Opthalmology,* 1974, *58,* 752-756.

Montgomery, J. D. Variations in perception of short time intervals during menstrual cycle. *Perceptual & Motor Skills,* 1979, *49,* 940-942.

Moos, R. *Menstrual Distress Questionnaire manual,* 1977. Social Ecology Laboratory, Department of Psychiatry and Behavioral Sciences, Stanford University, Palo Alto, CA 94305.

Moos, R. H. & Leiderman, D. B. Towards a menstrual cycle symptom typology. *Journal of Psychosomatic Research,* 1978, *22,* 31-40.

Morris, N. M. & Udry, J. R. Variations in pedometer activity during the menstrual cycle. *Obstetrics and Gynecology,* 1970, *35,* 199-201.

Most, A. F., Woods, N. F., Dery, G. K., & Most, B. M. Distress associated with menstruation among Israeli women. *International Journal of Nursing Studies,* 1981, *18,* 61-71.

Munchel, M. E. The effects of symptom expectations and response styles on cognitive and perceptual-motor performance during the menstrual phase. *Dissertation Abstracts International,* 1979, *39*(7-B), 3532.

Parlee, M. B. Menstruation and voluntary participation in a psychological experiment. Paper presented at the *Annual Meeting of the American Psychological Association*, Chicago, Illinois, 1975.

Pierson, W. R. & Lockhart, A. Effect of menstruation on simple reaction and movement time. *British Medical Journal*, 1963, *1*, 796-797.

Redgrove, J. A. Menstrual cycles. In W. P. Colquhoun (Ed.), *Biological rhythms and human performance*. London: Academic, 1971, 211-240.

Rodin, J. Menstruation, reattribution and competence. *Journal of Personality and Social Psychology*, 1976, *33*, 345-353.

Ruble, D. Premenstrual symptoms: A reinterpretation. *Science*, 1977, *197*(4300), 291-292.

Ruble, D. N. & Brooks-Gunn, J. Menstrual symptoms; a social cognition analysis. *Journal of Behavioral Medicine*, 1979, *2*, 171-194.

Schubert, G. W., Meyer, R. C., & Washer, S. H. Responses to short-duration signals, pre- and postmenses, in subjects using oral contraceptives and subjects not using oral contraceptives. *Journal of the American Audiological Society*, 1975, *1*, 112-118.

Schwank, J. C. H. The menstrual cycle and performance on various laboratory tasks. Unpublished manuscript, 1971.

Seward, G. H. Psychological effects of the menstrual cycle on women workers. *Psychological Bulletin*, 1944, *41*, 90-102.

Seward, G. H. *Sex and the social order*. New York: McGraw-HIll, 1946.

Silverman, E-M. & Zimmer, C. Speech fluency fluctuations during the menstrual cycle. *Journal of Speech and Hearing Research*, 1975, *18*, 202-206.

Silverman, E-M. & Zimmer, Ch. H. Replication of "speech fluency fluctuations during the menstrual cycle." *Perceptual & Motor Skills*, 1976, *42*, 1004-1006.

Slade, P. & Jenner, F. A. Performance tests in different phases of the menstrual cycle. *Journal of Psychosomatic Research*, 1980, *24*, 5-8.

Smith, A. J. Menstruation and industrial efficiency. I, Absenteeism and activity level. *Journal of Applied Psychology*, 1950a, *34*, 1-5.

Smith, A. J. Menstruation and industrial efficiency, II, Quality and quantity of production. *Journal of Applied Psychology*, 1950b, 34, 148-152.

Snyder, D. B. The relationship of the menstrual cycle to certain aspects of perceptual cognitive functioning. *Dissertation Abstracts International*, 1978, *39*(2-B), 962-963.

Sommer, B. Menstrual cycle changes and intellectual performance. *Psychosomatic Medicine*, 1972a, *34*, 263-269.

Sommer, B. Perceptual-motor performance, mood and the menstrual cycle. Paper presented at the *Annual Meeting of the Western Psychological Association*, Portland, Oregon, 1972b.

Sommer, B. The effect of menstruation on cognitive and perceptual-motor behavior: A review. *Psychosomatic Medicine*, 1973, *34*, 515-534.

Stenn, P. G. & Klinge, V. Relationship between the menstrual cycle and bodily activity in humans. *Hormones and Behavior*, 1972, *3*, 297-305.

Sugerman, A. A. et al. Quantitative EEG changes in the human menstrual cycle. *Research Communications in Chemical Pathology and Pharmacology*, 1970, *1*, 526-534.

Tedford, W. H., Warren, D. E., & Flynn, W. E. Alteration of shock aversion thresholds during the menstrual cycle. *Perception and Psychophysics*, 1977, *21*, 193-196.

The Tampax Report. Ruder Finn & Rotman, 110 E. 59th Street, New York, NY 10022.

Tuch, R. The relationship between a mother's menstrual status and her response to illness in her child. *Psychosomatic Medicine*, 1975, *37*, 388-394.

Uno, T. GSR activity and the human menstrual cycle. *Psychophysiology*, 1973, 10, 213-214.

Vierling, J. S. & Rock, J. Variations of olfactory sensitivity to Exaltolide during the menstrual cycle. *Journal of Applied Physiology*, 1967, *22*, 311-315.

Vila, J. & Beech, H. R. Vulnerability and defensive reactions in relation to the human menstrual cycle. *British Journal of Social and Clinical Psychology*, 1978, *17*, 93-100.

Vogel, W., Broverman, D. M., & Klaiber, E. L. EEG responses in regularly menstruating women and in amenorrheic women treated with ovarian hormones. *Science*, 1971, *172*, 388-391.

Walsh, R. N. Budtz-Olsen, I., Leader, C., & Cummins, R. A. The menstural cycle, personality, and academic performance. *Archives of General Psychiatry,* 1981, *38,* 219-221.

Ward, M. M., Stone, S. C., & Sandman, C. A. Visual perception in women during the menstrual cycle. *Physiology and Behavior,* 1978, *20,* 239-243.

Webster, S. K. Attributional approaches to the relationship of symptoms to cognitive performance across the menstrual cycle. *Dissertation Abstracts International,* 1979, *40*(6-B), 2909.

Wickham, M. The effects of the menstrual cycle on test performance. *British Journal of Psychology,* 1958, *49,* 34-41.

Wineman, E. W. Autonomic balance changes during the human menstrual cycle. *Psychophysiology,* 1971, *8,* 1-6.

Wong, S. & Tong, J. E. Menstrual cycle and contraceptive hormone effects on temporal discrimination. *Perceptual & Motor Skills,* 1974, *39,* 103-108.

Wright, P. & Crow, R. A. Menstrual cycle: Effect on sweetness preferences in women. *Hormones and Behavior,* 1973, *4,* 387-391.

Wuttke, W., Arnold, P., Becker, D., Creutzfeldt, O., Langenstein, S., & Tirsch, W. Hormonal profiles and variations of the EEG and of performances in psychological tests in women with spontaneous menstrual cycles and under oral contraceptives. In T. M. Itil (Ed.) *Psychotropic action of hormones.* New York: Spectrum Publications, 1976, 169-182.

Zimmerman, E. & Parlee, M. B. Behavioral changes associated with the menstrual cycle: An experimental investigation. *Journal of Applied Social Psychology,* 1973, *3,* 335-344.

Dysmenorrhea

Mary Anna Friederich, MD

ABSTRACT. Pain during the menstrual period is of two types: primary, in which the pelvic organs are normal and secondary, in which pathologic lesions are found on pelvic examination or laparoscopic examination of the pelvic organs. Since the incidence varies between 31-92% of the population it has serious implications for our society. It is important to distinguish dysmenorrhea from the premenstrual tension syndrome. Currently primary dysmenorrhea is thought to be due to increased contractility of the myometrium or decreased uterine blood flow from the excessive contractions or increased sensitization of pain fibers to mechanical and chemical stimuli. These three mechanisms of pain production are due to the release of certain prostoglandins from the endometrium during menses which then go directly into the myometrium producing these effects. Situational or psychological factors may accentuate or decrease the pain. Treatment is with antiprostoglandin drugs. There are several causes of secondary dysmenorrhea both congenital and acquired. Laparoscopy is frequently needed along with D&C to make the diagnosis. After diagnosis is made appropriate treatment can be undertaken to relieve the pain.

ACADEMIC AND ECONOMIC IMPLICATIONS

Several reseachers have studied the effect of dysmenorrhea on academic success and school adjustment in terms of the number of days lost from school due to dysmenorrhea. Again the percentages vary, but on the average between 10 and 14% of young women in their late teens and early 20's are absent from classes monthly because of dysmenorrhea (Klein & Litt, 1981; Morrison & Nicolls, 1981). Dysmenorrhea may affect the academic performance of women who do not absent themselves from school as well. Since academic success has long range implications for women who are training for their future occupations, dysmenorrhea may be a subtle influence on their futures.

The economic impact of dysmenorrhea is very difficult to assess.

It probably is under reported as a cause for loss of work. Many white collar workers may leave for the day without officially having to note the reason. Factory workers are more likely to have to record the reason. Many studies have been done on this, the most comprehensive being in the Scandinavian countries, Sweden and Norway. Their conclusion seems to be that dysmenorrhea as the cause of absence from work represents only a small portion of the total absences reported and working women do not lose more days due to illness per year than do men. However, women with significant dysmenorrhea do miss anywhere from 5-12 days more per year than do women with mild or no dysmenorrhea. Since more and more women are going into the work force, the impact was felt to be significant (Bergsjo, 1979; Svennerud, 1959). It is also impossible to estimate the loss of efficiency during working hours due to primary dysmenorrhea of women who do not leave work.

PREMENSTRUAL TENSION SYNDROME

Premenstrual tension syndrome refers to a group of symptoms usually occurring prior to the onset of menses. This can be anywhere from a few days to 10 days before. The symptoms include headache, irritability, depression, bloating, insomnia, painful breasts, and inability to concentrate. The premenstrual syndrome is very poorly understood. The severity and combination of symptoms varies from time to time and seem to be related to psychosocial factors as well as to physiology. Perhaps most important, however, are biochemical changes in neurotransmitters influencing the entire endocrine system about which we know nothing.

Of interest, the incidence of premenstrual tension is low in the teenage group but tends to increase in the 30 and 40 year old group (Golub, 1976, 1981; Moos, 1968).The important point here is that the premenstrual tension syndrome is a complex group of changes which should not be confused with dysmenorrhea.

PRIMARY DYSMENORRHEA

Clinical Features

The pain of primary dysmenorrhea characteristically starts a few hours before to 12 hours after the onset of flow and lasts about 24-36 hours. It is generally agreed that primary dysmenorrhea or dysmenorrhea associated with a completely normal pelvic examination is somehow related to ovulation. This association was first noted in 1938 by Wilson and Kurzrok (1938). Then Sturgis and Albright (1940) reported that estrogens when given sufficiently early in the cycle could suppress ovulation. Parental estrogen and later orally activate estrogen became mainstays in the treatment for severe dysmenorrhea. However, this was not a practical method to treat the problem because of the side effects of estrogen such as nausea, vomiting, and the irregular shedding which occurs after estrogen is withdrawn. It only became practical to suppress ovulation when oral progestins became available in the late 1950s. Primary dysmenor-rhea does not usually occur with menarche since menarche is anovulatory as are the first few cycles thereafter. The ovaries may take as long as 5 years to mature from the time of menarche. During those five years many cycles will be anovulatory. A typical history of a woman with primary dysmenorrhea is pain free menarche and pain free periods for one to two years, thereafter followed by the gradual onset of pain with periods which becomes increasingly severe in intensity and prolonged in duration. The pain is due to hypercontractility of the myometrium and resulting ischemia.

Myometrial Activity

The basic contractility pattern of the myometrium varies through-out the menstrual cycle according to the hormonal status of the uterus. Though the first successful experiment measuring non-pregnant uterine activity dates back to 1889 (Heinricius, 1889), it was not until the middle 1970s that microtransducers were available which markedly facilitated the accurate measurement of uterine pressures at different points in the uterus at the same time. Up to three microtransducers can be placed within the uterine cavity or cervical canal, making it possible to evaluate the propagation of a contraction wave. This was an improvement over previous tech-niques such as the microballoon and the open ended catheter which did not give exact reproducible pressures. And this new technology enabled us to learn more about uterine physiology.

The contractility pattern of the uterus varies in different phases of the menstrual cycle. During the proliferative phase there are fre-quent small contractions increasing to the highest frequency with a rise in tone around the time of ovulation. In the secretory phase there are fewer contractions with higher amplitudes developing to pre-labor-like activity before menstruation. Uterine contractility increases at menstruation and has been designated labor-like. It is characterized by contractions of higher amplitude and a regular frequency of about 3-10 per ten minutes. Most investigators agree that women with primary dysmenorrhea have a hypercontractile pattern. During severe cramps, extremely high amplitudes of 200-350 millimeters of mercury have been recorded. (Remember the highest pressure during the height of a labor contraction is 50 mm of mercury.) The frequency of contractions during dysmenorrhea is elevated to 6-12 every ten minutes as compared to 3-10 in normal cycles. A baseline tone ranging from 50-75 mm of mercury between contractions has been recorded in women with dysmenorrhea as well as asynchronous propagation of the waves. The hypercontractile state of the uterus results in a decrease in myometrial blood flow with ischemia which causes the pain.

Many factors affect the contractile pattern of the uterus. For example, sudden awakening from sleep will cause a strong, relatively short contraction lasting about 10 seconds but this only occurs during the secretory phase when the myometrium is under the influence of progestogens. Deep sleep on the other hand may cause relaxation of the uterine contractile pattern. If ovulation has not occurred, there are only the small frequent contractions of the proliferative phase during menstrual flow. If estrogens are administered to a menopausal woman or oophorectomized woman with sparce small contractions, a proliferative phase pattern will develop with more frequent small contractions. High doses of progestogens preceded by estrogen induce the frequent contractions of long duration and higher amplitude recognized as the secretory pattern.

Hormones

Primary dysmenorrhea is related to ovulatory cycles, yet the role of estrogens and progestins in the mechanism of dysmenorrhea still remains to be elucidated. Plasma estrogens and progesterone concentrations are not different in normal versus dysmenorrheic women. Urinary excretion studies are equivocal. Circulating levels do not necessarily reflect cellular endometrial and myometrial events. No information is available about steroid hormone receptor-binding activity in the myometrium and endometrium of dysmenorrheic women.

Oxytocin has an insignificant effect on the contractile pattern of the non-pregnant uterus whereas vasopressin is an effective uterine stimulant. Vasopressin decreases uterine blood flow both by increasing myometrial contractions and also by its direct effect on blood vessels. After intravenous injection, the minimum blood flow occurs considerably later than the maximal uterine activity (Akerlund & Andersson, 1976). Using radioimmunoassay, Akerlund (1979) demonstrated that the mean level of vasopressor concentration on day one of the cycle was double for dysmenorrheic woman as compared to controls. The high vasopressin level, however, may be the result of pain rather than the cause. Ethanol alleviates menstrual pain in part by causing vasodilatation, but also by inhibiting the central release of vasopressins.

Nothing is known about the levels of opiate receptors in the brain and β-endorphins, enkephalins, and other brain peptides in the circulation of women with primary dysmenorrhea.

Uterine Nerves

The uterus contains adrenergic and cholinergic nerves, but their involvement in the regulation of myometrial activity is not well understood. Presacral sympathectomy has been used to treat dysmenorrhea successfully in the past though there are few indications for its use now. Those nerves innervate both the smooth muscle cells and the uterine vascular bed. They originate in peripheral ganglion formations at the utero-vaginal junction and belong to a specific unit within the sympathetic nervous system called short adrenergic nerves. During pregnancy there is a marked progessive reduction of uterine adrenergic nerves. At term, only small amounts of noradrenaline can be measured in the uterus. The neurotransmitter loss is due to widespread nerve terminal degeneration. After delivery there is a regeneration of the sympathetic transmitter, but the noradrenaline concentration does not read pre-pregnant levels. This may account for the disappearance of dysmenorrhea following pregnancy (Sjöberz, 1979).

Prostaglandins

The concept of "toxins" in menstrual fluid dates back to antiquity, but it was not until the 1950s that Pickles (1957; 1959a, b; Pickles & Clitheroe, 1960) reported that the acetone extract from menstrual blood contained a substance that stimulated smooth muscle contractions. He termed the substance "menstrual stimulant" and postulated that it was produced in the endometrium. Thus began our knowledge of the importance of prostaglandins in menstrual cycle physiology. Prostaglandins are a group of endogenous substances which are 20-carbon hydroxy unsaturated fatty acids (prostanoic acid) with a cyclopentane ring and two side chains. There are many natural prostaglandins found in all tissues of the body. The ones most significant for the uterus are prostaglandins E_2 (PGE_2) and prostaglandin F_2 alpha ($PGF_{2\alpha}$). Prostaglandins are synthesized locally in tissues under the control of enzymes collectively called prostaglandin synthetases which are present in the microsomes of the cells. This very complicated biochemical process has been well outlined by Dawood (1981) in a recent summary article. Pickles was the first to demonstrate that the prostaglandins in the pooled menstrual fluid of dysmenorrheic patients was higher than in the menstrual fluid of non-dysmenorrheic women. Others have confirmed his observation both in menstrual fluid, and in uterine jet washings, and endometrial biopsies. Others have shown that circulating levels of some of the metabolic breakdown products of the $PGF_{2\alpha}$ are increased in dysmenorrheic women on the first day of the menses as compared to normal women but $PGF_{2\alpha}$ itself is not elevated in the peripheral circulation of women with dysmenorrhea compared to those without it. This is because $PGF_{2\alpha}$ is rapidly metabolized to 15-keto, 13, 14-dihydro-$PGF_{2\alpha}$. Eglinton and colleagues (1963) demonstrated that the endometrial content of $PGF_{2\alpha}$ and the ratio of $PGF_{2\alpha}$ to PGE_2 is higher during the secretory part of the menstrual cycle as compared to the proliferative stage. The synthesis of the prostaglandins in the endometrium though regulated by progesterone also involves several other factors—(1) the availability of precursor fatty acid (arachidonic acid), (2) estrogen, (3) epenephrine, (4) luteinizing hormone, (5) cellular trauma, (6) cyclic AMP. Exogenally administered PGE_2 and $PGF_{2\alpha}$ induce contractions of the myometrium in the non-pregnant woman. The contractions of the uterus previously described for normal and dysmenorrheic cycles are due to the cyclic production of prostaglandins. There is now strong evidence that women with dysmenorrhea produce more of these prostaglandins than do normal women. Such high concentrations may be due either to an increased production, abnormal release, or decreased breakdown. To date it has only been demonstrated that dysmenorrheic women do have an increased ability to synthesize prostaglandins from its precursor fatty acid arachidonic acid. As yet no good data are available on the production or metabolic clearance rates of PGE_2 and $PGF_{2\alpha}$ during menstruation.

The action of prostaglandins $PGF_{2\alpha}$ upon the myometrium depends upon both calcium and magnesium. Human myometrium has prostaglandin receptors. Prostaglandin $PGF_{2\alpha}$ acts at the myometrial cellular level to increase the influx of calcium across the myometrial cell membrane, and to block calcium binding to cytoplasmic membrane protein. The final result is to increase free calcium which triggers contractions of the myofibrils. By an unknown mechanism, prostaglandins may also deplete cellular magnesium. Magnesium causes depletion of ATP which leads to myometrial relaxation. Magnesium deficiency has been considered as a cause of dysmenorrhea.

At the end of the luteal phase of the menstrual cycle, the corpus luteum undergoes regression and progesterone production declines. Because less progesterone is reaching the endometrium, lysomes undergo breakdown and release enzymes which include phospholipases. These phopholipases act on the phospholipids in the cell membrane to generate arachidonic acid which is then available for prostaglandin synthesis. The production of PGE_2 and $PGF_{2\alpha}$ in the endometrium and their presence in the menstrual fluid lead to contraction of the myometrium. Why dysmenorrheic woman make excessive prostaglandins is unknown.

To summarize, there are three mechanisms by which prostaglandins produce menstrual pain. The first is through increased myometrial contraction. The second is by decreased uterine blood flow from the excessive contractions leading to ischemia. The third is through increased sensitization of pain fiber to mechanical and chemical stimuli such as bradykinin and histamine.

Psychological Considerations

Since menstruation is an outward and visible manifestation of a biologic process peculiar to woman, it is intimately associated with a woman's psychologic development from early childhood and her current psychosocial situation. Only the most unsophisticated clinician would maintain that dysmenorrhea is primarily psychogenic in origin. Once pain has been experienced, however, women will frequently become apprehensive as the next menses approaches. The expectation of pain may, indeed, induce more pain. Psychologic factors are definitely involved in the perception of any type of pain as evidenced by the fact that major surgery has been performed on people under hypnosis without any signs of pain. Following acute injury in battle, soldiers have shown no signs of pain. Pain is an unpleasant and very personal experience. It can not be objectively observed by another. All young women as they grow up have been exposed to cultural and familial expectations regarding menstruation including for some, the expectation of pain. Many cultures have had menstrual taboos indicating to the young woman that menstruation is a form of illness. To some extent this concept continues in our society today, i.e., the use of such terms for menses as "the curse," "falling off the roof," etc. Therefore, there is a complex interrelation between psychological and physiological factors of which the clinician needs to be aware in dealing with a given individual. As a rule of thumb, if the dysmenorrhea starts some months to years after menarche, has gradually increased in severity, and lasts approximately one day, it is most likely of a physiologic origin and is related to the prostaglandins. On the other hand, if the pain occurred with menarche and lasts more than one day, there is probably a psychological component. Some women may gather much secondary gain from seeing menstruation as an illness allowing them to rest from their usual activities and duties. Others may use illness as a way of denying the sexual and reproductive significance of the menstrual period. Many women are aware that at times of stress in their lives they have dysmenorrhea, whereas, at times of relative calm they do not have dysmenorrhea. If ovulation suppression and/or antiprostaglandin therapy does not help and a laparoscopy is normal, psychological problems should be considered.

Treatment

In seeing any woman with dysmenorrhea the clinician must take a good open-ended, non-directive history. A very good question to ask is "what do you remember about your first period." In this way the physician will learn about a very significant event in the life of the woman. Did she know about periods prior to her menarche? Who had told her about them? Was she able to talk with peers and mother about periods? Could she tell her mother and peers about her period when it arrived? In this way the physician will have some knowledge of a crucial time in psychobiologic development of this particular woman. The physician will also learn if the menarche was pain free and if the periods remained pain free for some time thereafter. It is also important to get a general medical history because certain debilitating illnesses may cause increasing symptoms of dysmenorrhea. While obtaining the history the physician is learning how much the pain interferes with the woman's everday activity. It may turn out that she comes for general reassurance and, indeed, is not too troubled by her symptoms. This will obviate giving of medication. Many woman can self medicate with over the counter drugs and just need to be reassured that their examination is normal. History of sexual activity is most important because it is not uncommon that certain woman will develop dysmenorrhea around the time they start sexual activity. Obviously while getting this history the physician can inquire about contraception. A general physical exam and careful pelvic exam are mandatory. After this history and physical examination, the physician will have an understanding of what type of treatment is indicated. As mentioned above, reassurance may be the only thing necessary for certain women. Certain others will need ovulation suppressants, particularly those needing contraception. Currently any of the low dose estrogen-progestin combinations taken from day 5 to day 25 of the cycle can be prescribed if the examination and the history are completely negative for pathology.

For women who do not need contraception or who would prefer not to suppress ovulation the prostaglandin synthetase inhibiting drugs are in order. There are many studies in the literature which show that about 80% of women are helped by these drugs. Sometimes if the first one does not work, switching to another will be helpful. These drugs are started at the first sign of menses. Originally they were started a day or two before, but if the woman might be pregnant this could be harmful to the fetus. There was no value in starting ahead of menstrual flow, so currently they are prescribed at onset of flow.

The exact mechanism of enzyme inhibition of these drugs is unknown. They preferentially inhibit the enzyme cyclo-oxygenase. This enzyme catalyzes the oxygenation and cyclization of arachidonic acid to form the cyclic endoperoxides which then undergo change to form the prostaglandins. Because the drugs block the initial steps in the metabolic pathway, these drugs act blindly and broadly. Their action is not restricted to the uterus.

There are 5 major groups of prostaglandin synthetase inhibitors:

1. Benzoic acid derivatives such as aspirin—this will help with mild pain. Dose: 500-650 mg., 4 times/day.
2. Buterophenones such as phenylbutazone—do not effectively inhibit cyclo-oxygenase.
3. Indole-acetic acid derivatives such as indomethacin. Usual dose: 25 mg., 3-6 times/day. This has high gastrointestinal side effects.
4. Fenamates—such as mefenamic acid. Usual dose: 250-500 mg., 3-4 times/day.
5. Arylpropionic acid derivatives such as: Ibuprofen 400 mg., 4 times/day; Naproxen sodium 275 mg., 4 times/day; Keto-profen 50 mg., twice a day.

If the original dose is not helpful, the starting dose may be increased by 50%, while keeping the maintenance dose the same. The woman takes this for as long as her pain usually lasts, i.e., 6-48 hours. Side effects include indigestion, heart burn, nausea, constipation, vomiting, diarrhea, headache, dizziness, vertigo, visual or hearing disturbances, drowsiness, skin rashes, bronchospasm, hematological abnormalities, and fluid retention. A definite contraindication is gastrointestinal ulcers. A relative contraindication is history of bronchospasm after ingesting aspirin.

Calcium antagonists may become available shortly for use by woman who are not helped by the antiprostaglandin drugs. As mentioned previously, an influx of free calcium into the cells causes contractions of the myofibrils. Calcium antagonists prevent this influx. Nifedipine is one of the most potent calcium antagonists used in one in vivo study. Uterine contractile patterns showed rapid relaxation 15 minutes after oral intake of 30 mg. of the drug. However, there are side effects, such as flushing and headaches, which have not made it feasible for this to become a routine treatment.

Beta$_2$ receptor stimulating drugs are also a possibility after these drugs have been refined. Intravenous administration of terbutaline, the beta$_2$ receptor stimulatory agent, instantly suppressed uterine activity in dysmenorrheic women much more effectively than the prostaglandin inhibitors. However, due to the side effects of these drugs, which include tremor, tachycardia, and palpitations, they are not acceptable yet in the management of severe dysmenorrhea.

If ovulation suppression or antiprostaglandin drugs are not helpful the next step should be diagnostic laparoscopy since a certain number of women will be found to have small amounts of endometriosis or evidence of pelvic inflammatory disease to account for their dysmenorrhea. Even teenagers will have these findings. Dilation of the cervix sometimes gives temporary relief of primary dysmenorrhea. Curettage may rule out intrauterine pathology. Presacralneurectomy or removal of the autonomic nerves to the uterus is rarely used now. Indeed, most insurance plans will not pay for it.

Women with a history of primary dysmenorrhea are not good candidates for intrauterine devices because the IUD may only increase their pain. However, the progestasert intrauterine device which releases small amounts of progesterone may be used and may decrease pain.

SECONDARY DYSMENORRHEA

Congenital and Acquired

Secondary dysmenorrhea can be divided into congenital and acquired. Causes include such conditions as a congenital blind pouch of the uterus which may be lined with endometrium that cycles and sheds but from which, since there is no opening, the flow can not escape; thus, pressure builds up and pain occurs. This pain may be colicky in nature starting near the menarche and occurring towards the end of the menstrual period rather than at the beginning as in primary dysmenorrhea. Congenital imperforate hymen may also cause dysmenorrhea by producing hematocolpos. Acquired causes of dysmenorrhea include submucous myomas, endometrial or endocervical polyps, endometriosis, adenomyosis, acute and chronic pelvic inflammatory disease, presence of an intrauterine device, or cervical stenosis. History is most important in the diagnosis of secondary dysmenorrhea. The pain is less characteristically related to first day of flow than with primary dysmenorrhea and may be present for some time before or after the actual menses. Patients with secondary dysmenorrhea tend to be older than those with primary. Pain tends to be progressive with age rather than decreasing with age as with primary. Careful general physical and pelvic examinations are obviously important in making the diagnosis.

Laparoscopy is frequently needed, particularly in the case of endometriosis.

Endrometriosis

Etiology and incidence. Endometriosis is a non-malignant condition in which the endometrium or lining of the uterus appears to implant in the pelvis, abdomen, abdominal wall, or chest. There are two possible etiologies—one, that fragments of endometrium regurgitate through the fallopian tubes and implant in the peritoneal cavity. This, however, does not explain why endometriosis can appear at distant sites such as the thorax and the skin of the abdominal wall. However, TeLinde and Scott (1950) did show in rhesus monkeys that if the cervix was occluded the monkeys menstruated through their tubes and developed endometriosis foci in the pelvis. Similar foci have also been reported in men. This points to a more encompassing theory, namely that of coelomic metaplasia. This theory postulates that the coelomic epithelium is multi-potential and can undergo endometrial metaplasia when properly stimulated.

Endometriosis may be extensive in the abdomen and pelvis without any signs or symptoms. On the other hand it may account for dysmenorrhea and infertility. In Sampson's (1927) original report, approximately 50% of the patients with endometriosis complained of dysmenorrhea and these statistics have held up in later reports. The incidence of endometriosis appears to be increasing, probably because gynecologists are doing more laparoscopies and because woman are waiting longer to conceive. Because women are having more menstrual periods, there are more opportunities for endometrium to reflux out of the tubes and settle in the pelvis. It used to be thought that endometriosis didn't appear until after 10 or more years of menstruation, but more recently it has been found in teenage women. Some have estimated that a third of patients presenting with pelvic pain and infertility will have endometriosis. There is a clear familial incidence. Women who have a first degree relative affected by endometriosis have a seven times higher risk of developing it than woman who have no such affected relative. Approximately one third of all women with severe endometriosis are likely to have an affected first degree relative. The genetic mechanism is not understood. It was formerly believed that this disease affects whites more than blacks but this has more recently been refuted.

Clinical features. Patients who have dysmenorrhea associated with endometriosis complain of progressively severe acquired dysmenorrhea. Usually the pain is located in the lower abdomen bilaterally and associated with rectal pressure. However, the pain can be unilateral since the pain relates to the shedding of the endometrium in the implant. If implants are on one side of the pelvis, the pain will be felt on that side. Pain may start premenstrually and continue throughout the entire length of the period. Intercourse frequently makes the pain worse as does defecation. If there are endometrial implants in the subplural region the patient may complain of constricting substernal chest pain, shortness of breath, and shoulder pain at the onset of a period. A chest x-ray will reveal evidence of a pneumothorax. Why all women with endometriosis do not have pain is unknown. A significant increase of $PGF_{2\alpha}$ has been found in the peritoneal fluid of patients with endometriosis as compared to that of control subjects. And increased concentrations of PGE_2 and $PGF_{2\alpha}$ have been found in the endometrium of patients with endometriosis as well. The administration of prostaglandin antagonists can partially, if not completely, relieve pelvic pain associated with endometriosis. Some women with mild endometriosis are infertile. This is often hard to explain if the fallopian tubes are patent. Again, infertility has been attributed to prostaglandin increases but this has yet to be completely understood.

The diagnosis is often strongly suspected on clinical grounds. Some women have the classic pelvic examination of a fixed retroverted uterus, distinct nodular thickening of the utero sacral ligaments, and adnexal masses adhered to the lateral pelvic wall. On the other hand with very early endometriosis, the patient will have a normal pelvic exam and the gynecologist will have to do a laparoscopy in order to confirm the diagnosis. A biopsy should always be done of the implants if at all possible since there are other types of implants, such as spleenosis, which can resemble endometriosis.

Treatment. Once the diagnosis has been made, the choice of therapy depends upon the age of the patient, her desire for conception, the severity of her symptoms, and the extent of the disease. For instance, if the disease has caused obstruction of the bowel, radical surgery removing the ovaries may be necessary to prevent the continued cycling of the endometriosis. On the other hand, observation and symptomatic treatment may be sufficient for a patient with mild endometriosis with mild symptoms who does not plan to conceive immediately. It is wise to advise such a woman that if she puts off conception her chances will be greatly reduced. No treatment can prevent endometriosis or selectively destroy the ectopic endometrium and, therefore, cure the disease. The only method which assures a permanant cure is castration. All other methods are temporary at best.

There are two forms of medical management currently. The first is so-called pseudo-pregnancy in which the woman takes increasingly large doses of estrogen and progesterone to stop the cycling. It is the ovarian cycling that keeps the implants growing. Exogenous sex steroids suppress gonadotrophin secretions thereby inhibiting ovarian function. The dose starts as low as possible but then gradually must be increased because of breakthrough bleeding from the uterine endometrium. This in continued for anywhere from 6-12 months depending upon the extent of the disease and the improvement during the treatment. Many women get side effects of bloating, weight gain, and/or breakthrough bleeding and, therefore, are not too pleased with this regime. Indeed, only about 50% can tolerate a complete course of treatment because of the side effects. Overall pregnancy rates following this treatment have reported to be as high as 50% by some researchers. Recurrence after treatment usually occurs. The second type of medical therapy is pseudomenopause, again suppressing the gonadotrophins and producing a hypo-estrogenic state in order to cause regression of the implants. Danazol, a synthetic steroid with antigonadotrophic properties, is given. Danazol is related to 17 alpha ethinyl testosterone and as such is mildly androgenic and anabolic. It acts either on the pituitary or the hypothalamus and perhaps directly on the ovary and the endometrium. Blood estrogen and progesterone levels are those of the early follicular phase of the normal cycle. Side effects include: atropic vaginitis, hot flashes, night sweats, hirsutism, weight gain, and acne. The daily dose is 800 mgm. a day for 3-9 months. This is a rather expensive drug. Symptomatic improvement has been reported in anywhere from 70-94% of patients with improvement in the pelvic findings in about 80% of treated patients. Menstruation returns 4-6 weeks after discontinuing the therapy. The pregnancy rate following treatment ranges from 83% in mild endometriosis to 38% in patients with severe endometriosis. The drug is largely used in infertility patients rather than for control of symptoms.

Surgical management of endometriosis can be either conservative or definitive, definitive meaning removing uterus, tubes, and both ovaries. The latter is done when the woman is having severe symptoms and has completed her family. Some authors feel that conservative surgery, i.e., removing the implants, has a better success rate as far as pregnancy goes than does medical therapy. This is still a controversial matter. The uterus may be suspended at the time of conservative surgery to keep the salpinx out of the pelvis where most of the implants are likely to occur. The incidence of conception following conservative surgery has been as high as 75% but as low as 38%. In one study, 47% of patients who had conservative surgery required repeat operations after 2 years of follow-up because of symptoms. This depends more on the original extent of the disease than it does on the type of surgery done.

The physician can review the various methods of therapy with each individual patient, explaining the various options, and involving her in the decision making process.

REFERENCES

Akerlund, M., & Andersson, K.E. Vasopressin response and terbutaline inhibition of the uterus. *Obstetrics & Gynecology,* 1976, *48,* 528.

Akerlund, M. Pathophysiology of dysmenorrhea. *Acta Obstetricia et Gynecologica Scandinavica. Supplement,* 1979, *87,* 27.

Bergsjo, P. Socioeconomic implications of dysmenorrhea. *Acta Obstetricia et Gynecologica Scandinavica. Supplement,* 1979, *87,* 67.

Dawood, M.Y. Hormones, prostaglandins, and dysmenorrhea. In M.Y. Dawood (Ed.) *Dysmenorrhea.* Baltimore: Williams & Wilkins, 1981.

Eglinton, G., Raphael, R.A., Smith, G.N., Hall W.J., & Pickles, U.R. Isolation and identification of two smooth muscle stimulants from menstrual fluid. *Nature,* 1963, *200,* 960.

Golub, S. The magnitude of premenstrual anxiety and depression. *Psychosomatic Medicine,* 1976, *38,* 4-12.

Golub, S. Premenstrual and menstrual mood changes in adolescent women. *Journal of Personality and Social Psychology,* 1981, *41,* 961-965.

Heinricius, G. En metod att grafiskt atergive kontradtioner hos en icke gravid livmoder. *Finska, Lakarsallskapets Handlingar,* 1889, *31,* 349.

Klein, J.R. & Litt, I.F. Epidemiology of adolescent dysmenorrhea. *Pediatrics,* 1981, *68,* 661.

Lamb, E.J. Clinical features of primary dysmenorrhea. In M.Y. Dawood (Ed.) *Dysmenorrhea.* Baltimore: Williams & Wilkins, 1981.

Moos, R. Development of a menstrual distress questionnaire. *Psychosomatic Medicine,* 1968, *30,* 853.

Morrison, J.C. & Nicholls, E.T. Epidemiologic, social, and economic aspects of dysmenorrhea. In M.Y. Dawood (Ed.) *Dysmenorrhea.* Baltimore: Williams & Wilkins, 1981.

Pickles, V.R. A plain-muscle stimulant in the menstruum. *Nature,* 1957, *180,* 1198.

Pickles, V.R. Some evidence that the human endometrium produces a hormone that stimulates plain muscle. *Journal of Endocrinology,* 1959a, *18,* 1.

Pickles, V.R. Myometrial responses to the menstrual plain-muscle stimulant. *Journal of Endocrinology,* 1959b, *19,* 150.

Pickles, V.R. & Clitheroe, H.J. Further studies of the menstrual stimulant. *Lancet,* 1960, *2,* 959.

Sampson, J.A. Peritoneal endometriosis due to menstrual dissemination of endometrial tissue into the peritoneal cavity. *American Journal of Obstetrics and Gynecology*, 1927, *14*, 442.

Sjoberz, N. Dysmenorrhea and uterine neurotransmitters. *Acta Obstetricia et Gynecologica Scandinavica. Supplement*, 1979, *87*, 27.

Sturgis, S.H. & Albright, F. The mechanism of estrin therapy in the relief of dysmenorrhea. *Endocrinology*, 1940, *26*, 68.

Svennerud, S. Dysmenorrhea and absenteeism. *Acta Obstetricia et Gynecologica Scandinavica. Supplement 2*, 1959, *38*, 1.

TeLinde, R.W. & Scott, R.D. Experimental endometriosis. *American Journal of Obstetrics and Gynecology* 1950, *60*, 1147.

Wilson, L. & Kurzrok, R. Studies on the motility of the human uterus in vivo. A functional myometrial cycle. *Endocrinology*, 1938, *23*, 79.

Premenstrual Syndrome:
A Selective Review

Judith M. Abplanalp, PhD

ABSTRACT. This review considers premenstrual syndrome (PMS) from the point of view of definitional issues, treatment issues, and the impact of the recent popularization of the syndrome. With respect to definition, problems include the lack of a consensus among researchers and clinicians concerning number, combination, and variety of symptoms, time cause, criteria for patient/subject selection, relationship of psychiatric disorder(s) to PMS, and determination of the existence of several PMS syndromes vs. one syndrome. Given the problems with definition, recommendations about appropriate treatment are difficult. Most treatment trials have lacked adequate controls for evaluation of placebo effects. The popularization of PMS but the mass media has raised collective consciousness about the syndrome but may also have raised hopes prematurely for a "cure."

The premenstrual syndrome (PMS) has intrigued investigators from many disciplines. Because the symptoms are both psychological and physiological, and because the menstrual cycle is itself a biological phenomenon, researchers from the the biological as well as the social sciences have contributed to the PMS research literature. The following areas of interest have been investigated most intensively:

1. Pathophysiology: e.g., (a) The relationship between levels of ovarian hormones or the ratios between them and premenstrual symptomatology; (b) The role of fluid retention in the appearance and magnitude of symptoms;
2. The relationship between cultural beliefs about the menstrual cycle and occurrence of premenstrual symptoms;

3. The relationship between PMS and psychiatric disorder; and the relationship between personality traits and PMS;
4. The role of stress in the production or exacerbation of premenstrual complaints;
5. Definition of PMS;
6. Assessment of PMS;
7. Treatment modalities for PMS and the theoretical bases for selection of treatment;
8. Etiology of PMS.

This paper includes a selective review of just two of these areas (Definition and Treatment) and a consideration of one additional content area (PMS in the recent popular literature).

The choice of topics was guided by a desire to present material which is central to the study of PMS in a way that would offer understandable information to the neophyte but would not be overly repetitious for the reader well versed in this literature.

Several reviews are recommended for the reader who wishes to pursue additional information on some of the other content areas. These are:

TOPIC	*SOURCE*
1. Pathophysiology, etiology (esp. physiological)	Reid and Yen (1981)
2. Stress	Abplanalp, Haskett & Rose (1980) Sommer (1978)
3. Psychiatric Disorder	Abplanalp, Haskett & Rose (1980) Clare (1982)
4. Assessment	Abplanalp, Haskett & Rose (1980) Sampson & Prescott (1981)
5. Treatment	Clare (1979) Reid and Yen (1981) Steiner & Carroll (1977)

TOPIC	SOURCE
6. Definition	Abplanalp, Haskett & Rose (1980) Parlee (1973)
7. Etiology	Abplanalp, Haskett & Rose (1980) Parlee (1973) Ruble & Brooks-Gunn (1979) Smith (1975)

DEFINITION

At first glance, it may seem unnecessary to devote one substantial section of this paper to the issue of definition. After all, the term ''premenstrual syndrome'' would appear to denote a certain cluster of symptoms which are time-locked to the menstrual cycle in a certain way. However, the matter is, in fact, more complicated.

With respect to premenstrual syndrome, the number and variety of symptoms may vary widely from one study to another, from one woman to another, and within the same woman, from one cycle to another. There does seem to be a common, If frequently unarticulated agreement, that symptoms may include emotional, somatic, and behavioral components.

The emotional states most commonly reported in studies of PMS are tension, anxiety, depression, irritability, and hostility. Somatic complaints include abdominal bloating, swelling, breast tenderness, headache, and backache. Behavioral changes frequently reported are an avoidance of social contact, a change in work habits, increased tendency to pick fights (especially with spouse/partner or children), and crying spells.

These examples, however, represent only a sampling of the symptoms which may be mentioned in connection with PMS. The number of potential items in each category is very large; and the three categories already mentioned (emotional, somatic, and behavior change) do not constitute an exhaustive list of those possible. Changes in appetite (e.g., specific food cravings or avoidance of certain foods), changes in sexual feelings (increase or decrease in libido) or behavior, and changes in motor coordination (more household accidents, difficulty in sports such as tennis) are also mentioned as part of the premenstrual syndrome.

There is, therefore, no one set of symptoms which is considered to be the hallmark of or standard criterion for defining the premenstrual syndrome.

The question of onset, and time course of the symptoms is equally problematic. At issue here is the fact that the term "premenstrual" means different things to different investigators.

To some extent the definition of the premenstrual syndrome is determined by the exigencies of the experimental design. If an investigator collects data only on the one day preceding the onset of menses, then the results of the study obviously cannot speak to the issue of development of symptomatology during the premenstrual phase. If the investigator inquires about the differences in emotional states throughout the menstrual cycle but does not collect information concerning the intensity of the moods, then the results do not address the question of severity of changes at different cycle phases.

Naturally, no one investigation can study all aspects of PMS. The point, however, is that the variables selected for study by an investigator reflect the researcher's beliefs about which variables are important; and some methodologies are inherently easier to implement than others. In the absence of a consensually agreed upon defintion of the syndrome, experimental designs often evolve from a combination of the experimenter's philosophy and his/her familiarity with certain methodological precedures. In effect, on some occasions the methodology appears to receive primary consideration, and the questions are posed second, thus reversing the "normal" order of the scientific method.

Of course, even if all researchers agreed on "the" definition of PMS, the methodological difficulties discussed above would not necessarily disappear.

However, a clearly stated consensually agreed-upon definition would, at least, increase the probability that comparisons between studies (which are very difficult at present) would be possible and valid because (a) different investigators would use similar inclusionary and exclusionary criteria for the selection of subjects, and (b) the criteria for defining the onset and duration of the premenstrual phase would be constant across studies.

We have elsewhere (Abplanalp et al., 1980) listed several factors which should be taken into consideration in the task of attempting to define PMS. These include: (1) the number and combination of symptoms; (2) severity; (3) time course (on-off characteristics, duration) of symptoms; (4) age of subjects/patients; (5) evaluation of validity of sources of information for assessment of the symptomatology.

The reader is referred to the earlier publication for a discussion of the importance of each factor.

Two additional factors which should be added to this list are (1) history of psychiatric illness and (2) evaluation of current psychological state (i.e., presence or absence of ongoing psychological/psychiatric problems).

Another aspect of the controversy surrounding the issue of the definition question of whether it is appropriate to speak of "the" premenstrual syndrome, or whether there are in fact, several premenstrual syndromes. A review of the PMS literature reveals that in most of the studies which have been published, there is an assumption, albeit frequently implicit, that there is but one premenstrual syndrome. Operationally this has meant that all symptoms, regardless of origin, are given equal weight. Thus, three subjects in a study of PMS may complain, respectively, of somatic symptoms only (e.g., abdominal bloating and breast tenderness), of emotional symptoms only (e.g., irritability and depression), or of a combination of symptoms (e.g., headaches and anxiety), and data from each woman would be treated as equivalent. In such cases, the researchers seem to be assuming that "a" premenstrual syndrome exists as an entity, but that it may take many different forms. As discussed above, the issue of severity of symptomatology is often not addressed at all. Thus, the same label, e.g., "premenstrual depression," may refer both to women who feel a bit sad during the premenstrual phase and to women who are clinically depressed and suicidal premenstrually.

In the past few years, several investigators have attempted to define PMS using more stringent criteria than has usually been the case, in order to document the presence of a more or less "pure" premenstrual syndrome. In theory, this term "pure" refers to the presence of symptoms premenstrually which are absent at all other times during the menstrual cycle. In practice, however, given the nature of the most commonly reported symptoms (e.g., tension, anxiety, irritability), PMS really refers to a significant *increase* during the premenstrual phase.

As Clare (1980, 1981) has pointed out, the symptoms which make up the syndrome are not uncommon "and occur intermittently in women of childbearing years . . . . In such cases, only the evidence of a premenstrual exacerbation of symptoms occurring at other times may indicate a premenstrual component'' (1981, p. 83).

Within the past few years, some investigators have begun to articulate more clearly and precisely criteria for inclusion in studies of PMS. This represents, hopefully, the beginning of an encouraging trend.

The criteria applied in the study by Haskett et al. (1980) and Steiner et al. (Note 4) were: (1) premenstrual dysphoric symptoms for at least six preceding menstrual cycles; (2) moderate to severe physical *and* psychological premenstrual symptoms; (3) symptoms *only* during the premenstrual period with marked *relief at onset of* menses; (4) age between 18 and 45 years; (5) not pregnant; (6) no hormonal contraception; (7) regular menses for six previous cycles; (8) no psychiatric disorder, normal physical examination and laboratory test profile; (9) no drugs for preceding four weeks; (10) will not receive the following drugs during the study: anxiolitics, diuretics, hormones, neuroleptics.

As is frequently the case when stringent criteria are employed, 5 out of 6 volunteers who requested to participate in this ''premenstrual tension syndrome'' study did not qualify.

In another recent study (Abplanalp, Note 1; Note 2; Haskett & Abplanalp, Note 3) similar selection criteria were employed, and in this study, again only 20% of those who volunteered met all the criteria for participation in the research.

Voluntary attrition was rare in these studies. The most common reasons for involuntary attrition were: (1) symptoms too mild to qualify (e.g., mood change but no associated changes in behavior); (2) symptoms present and of equivalent intensity at several points throughout the menstrual cycle; and (3) presence of psychiatric disorder (e.g., ongoing depressive symptomatology, not limited to premenstrual phase).

For some researchers, PMS is seen as several different syndromes, each consisting of a cluster of symptoms. The methodology employed by investigators with this view usually (though not always) involves the use of factor analytic techniques with data from large subject populations. This philosophy is reflected in the collaborative efforts of Endicott and Halbreich (Endicott et al., 1981; Halbreich & Endicott, 1982; Halbreich et al., 1982) and in the work of Abraham (1980) and Moos and Leiderman (1978).

One advantage of this approach is that it permits the researcher to examine PMS within a larger context than is possible with the smaller, more intensive studies described above. Thus, Endicott and Halbreich, in their work, have studied the relationship of premenstrual symptoms to psychiatric (especially affective) disorders. Subjects in these studies may be selected on the basis of criteria other than their premenstrual symptomatology. This avoids the kind of bias inherent in menstrual cycle research when subjects are aware of the purpose of the study.

On the other hand, although the presence of some premenstrual symptoms is fairly common among women, the existence of severe debilitating PMS is apparently relatively rare. Thus, when largely unselected subject samples are employed, the probability that the investigator will, by chance, collect a sufficient number of women to study severe PMS is quite small.

Once again because of the lack of consensually agreed upon definition(s) each investigator's assumptions about what constitutes PMS becomes important. We don't know, for example, whether the severe, disabling premenstrual symptoms reported by a relatively few women represent one end of a continuum, which also includes the much milder forms of the same symptoms reported by many women. The issue has not been addressed, in part because we don't have well-developed criteria for external validation of the syndrome(s).

The underlying assumption of most workers in PMS research is that this is a biologically based disorder. For investigators who adopt the multi-syndrome approach, the ability to differentiate between different clusters of symptoms on a statistical basis offers the hope that such a separation may eventually clarify etiological questions and may be instrumental in implementing different approaches to treatment and patient management.

It is important to note, however, that the multifactorial approach to defining premenstrual syndromes is in its infancy. The clinical advantage of the statistically derived symptom clusters or subtypes remains to be established, as does the usefulness of the subgroups with respect to selection of treatment modality.

In summary, it is clear that the issue of definition in PMS research is extremely important. On the other hand, it does not appear as though investigators are ready to come to an agreement about definition, for many question remain in exploratory stages. Thus, perhaps the best we can hope for at this point is to underscore the importance of complete communication of methodological approaches in published studies of PMS. The inclusionary and exclusionary criteria for subject selection should be discussed in detail. These should contain clear descriptions of the following: (1) specification of the ways in which subjects were recruited; (2) age limitations; (3) contraception and medication information; (4) marital status; (5) parity; (6) race; (7) menstrual history data; (8) assessment instruments; (9) operational definition of PMS; (10) psychiatric history data; (11) assessment of current psychological state; (12) criteria for assessment of severity of symptoms; (13) criteria for defining ovulatory status of cycle; (14) cut-off criteria for "unacceptable" subjects.

At the very least, such an improvement in communication will permit more valid evaluation of individual studies than has been possible to date. And hopefully, on a more optimistic note, the increased possibilities for replication which will result from more complete methodological descriptions will lead eventually to better clarification of factors necessary to reach a consensus about definition.

TREATMENT

There have been, over the past 50 years, ever since Frank's (1931) original description of the syndrome, a large number of published reports describing a wide variety of different treatments for alleviation of the symptoms related to PMS.

For example, PMS has been treated with oral contraceptives (combination estrogen and progesterone pills) (Cullberg, 1972; Smith, 1975); estrogen alone; natural progesterone (Dalton, 1964; 1977); synthetic progestogens (O'Brien et al., 1980; Sampson, 1979); valium and other minor tranquilizers; nutritional supplements (e.g., pyridoxine); minerals (magnesium, calcium); lithium; diuretics (e.g., bumetanid, sprionolactone); a prolactin inhibitor/dopamine agonist, bromocriptine; exercise; and psychotherapy (including relaxation, education, reassurance).

Three recent reviews (Clare, 1979; Reid & Yen, 1981; Steiner & Carroll, 1977) attest to the quantity of the treatment literature and also underscore the need for better quality of research designs. The interested reader is referred to these sources for comprehensive discussions of the relative effectiveness of the various treatments.

The majority of treatment studies in this area of research have involved open, uncontrolled trials, which do not permit accurate assessment of the treatment under consideration. In the relatively few studies which involved double-blind evaluation of a treatment agent and a placebo it has been obvious that significant placebo effects are commonplace in PMS (Sampson, 1979; Tonks, 1975). This means that almost anything used for treatment will be perceived as effective—helpful—to a certain proportion of the women participating in the "treatment" trial. Thus, as Elsner et al. (1980) have stated: "Open and/or uncontrolled trials do not provide adequate evaluation of new treatments for PMT. Controls for placebo effects are essential because women with PMT benefit from treatment regardless of what is used" (p. 723).

Sampson (1979) conducted one of the few double-blind controlled trials of the effectiveness of progesterone in the treatment of PMS. The results of the study suggested that placebo was at least as effective as progesterone. Sampson (1981a) subsequently commented:

> Uncontrolled studies or reports from clinics suggest that progesterone is helpful in premenstrual syndrome. When reviewing the treatment of premenstrual syndrome by any therapy given in an uncontrolled study one finds impressive results. However, when the treatment is given in a controlled double-blind study there is usually (a) a high placebo response and (b) the active agent is usually no better than a placebo. (p. 56)

Historically, each new treatment has been presented by its authors with a great deal of enthusiasm. None of the treatments, however, has *unequivocally* withstood the test of double-blind controlled trials (Steiner & Carroll, 1977). The recent discussions (controversy) on the role of prolactin in PMS and the use of bromocriptine (a prolactin inhibitor/dopamine agonist) in the treatment of the syndrome provide a good illustration of this phenomenon.

A relationship between prolactin and the symptoms of PMS was first proposed by Horrobin (1973). Subsequently, Halbreich et al. (1976) reported that prolactin levels were significantly higher through the menstrual cycle in PMS subjects than in asymptomatic women. At about the same time, Benedek-Jaszmann and Hearn-Sturtevant (1976) reported successful treatment of PMS in 10 women who participated in a double-blind crossover trial of bromocriptine and placebo. Bromocriptine seemed to be effective in alleviating all symptoms assessed. The results demonstrated quite dramatically that bromocriptine suppressed prolactin levels. On the other hand, prolactin values during the placebo cycles did not appear to be abnormally high.

Benedek-Jaszmann and Hearn-Sturtevant were so enthusiastic about these findings that they wrote: "We believe we may have found the key to the aetiology of the syndrome" (1976, p. 1096).

Other investigators, however, were not so convinced. Ghose and Coppen (1977) in a double-blind crossover design found no difference between bromocriptine and placebo on PMS symptom scores. There were several methodological problems with this study, however, in that: prolactin levels were not reported; the procedure for rating of symptoms is unclear; and the symptom scores are reported as a single, summed value, thus possibly obscuring real changes in individual symptoms.

Graham, Harding, Wise, and Berriman (1978), in another double-blind crossover bromocriptine-vs.-placebo study, reported significant improvement in "most" PMS symptoms during the bromocriptine cycles only. However, symptom data were reported for only the last 5 days of each cycle, thus making it impossible to determine to what extent symptoms were truly "premenstrual." Additionally, the absolute levels reported for anxiety, depression, etc., were low even during the placebo cycle.

Andersen et al. (1977) found that subjective complaints (e.g., headache, irritability, edema, abdominal distention, mastodynia) were decreased during both placebo and bromocriptine cycles in a double-blind crossover study. In fact, however, the only symptom which was *significantly* more improved by bromocriptine than by placebo was mastodynia (pain in the breast), which is not one of the more common PMS symptoms. As in the earlier research, bromocriptine was an effective suppressor of prolactin levels. However, again, there was no evidence that prolactin levels were elevated to begin with.

Andersch et al. (1978a; 1978b; 1979) compared the effects of bromocriptine and a diuretic (bumetanid) on prolactin levels and on premenstrual somatic and psychological symptoms. Both bromocriptine and the diuretic appeared to be beneficial in effecting symptom reduction. However, it is difficult to evaluate the relative effectiveness or either drug in this study, as neither the symptomatic subjects nor the asymptomatic controls received a placebo trial.

Elsner et al. (1980) subsequently demonstrated directly the power of placebo effects in a bromocriptine-placebo study. The group given "placebo only" reported significant improvement in premenstrual ratings of several symptoms. In fact, bromocriptine was superior to placebo on only three of the eight symptoms for which subjects kept daily records.

In their review of the role of prolactin in the etiology of premenstrual dysphoria, Carroll and Steiner (1978) proposed that PMS resulted from an interaction between a combination of either high levels of prolactin with low levels of estrogen (producing premenstrual depression) or high levels of prolactin with low levels of progesterone (producing premenstrual anxiety/irritability).

However, with the exception of the study by Halbreich et al. (1976), most investigators have reported that prolactin levels in women with PMS are within normal limits. Even Backstrom and his collaborators (Backstrom & Carstensen, 1974; Backstrom & Mattson, 1975; Backstrom et al., 1976; Backstrom et al., 1981) who have repeatedly asserted that PMS is related to levels and/or ratios of the ovarian hormones (estrogen and progesterone) recently assessed prolactin levels (Backstrom & Aakvaag, 1981) and found no difference between PMS subjects and controls.

Furthermore, subsequent to their reviews of PMS and the potential role of prolactin (Steiner & Carroll, 1977; Carroll & Steiner, 1978), the enthusiasm of these researchers was considerably dampened by their own study. In a carefully designed double-blind experiment whose purpose in part was to assess the effectiveness of bromocriptine on severe PMS, Steiner et al. (Note 4) found that 70-80% of the subjects both in the placebo and in the three treatment groups reported equivalent and significant relief of symptoms.

REVIEW OF POPULAR LITERATURE

During the past few years, both dysmenorrhea (severe pain with menses) and premenstrual syndrome have become topics discussed everywhere from TV talk shows to dinner tables across America. In large part, this shedding of the taboo against open public discussion of events connected with the menstrual cycle is a function of two factors, one concerning dysmenorrhea and the other relating to PMS. First was the discovery that symptoms of dysmenorrhea may result from overabundance of prostaglandins premenstrually which act in the uterus to produce strong contractions and associated severe pain. The development of synthetic drugs which act to reduce prostaglandin activity subsequently revolutionized the treatment of dysmenorrhea. In providing for the medical community a physiological explanation as well as a physiologically based treatment, dysmenorrhea became, apparently overnight, "acceptable" as a medical problem. The publication and subsequent publicity of a book written by a physician and designed to translate the scientific findings concerning the anti-prostaglandin research into language understandable to the lay public (Budoff, 1980) served as a powerful vehicle to legitimize open discussion of menstruation. It would be difficult, after all, to maintain a cloud of secrecy surrounding the topic when millions of Americans watched and listened to the subject of menstrual cramps being discussed on a TV talk show while they drank their morning cup of coffee.

In England, within the past year, in separate trials, several women accused of murder received probated or reduced sentences on the grounds that they suffered from a severe form of premenstrual syndrome which rendered them prone to uncontrollable acts of aggression during the week or so before the onset of menstruation (when the crimes for which each was being tried had been committed). The defense attorneys argued in these cases that at the time of the trial, the women were no longer a danger to society because effective treatment enabled them to live symptom-free lives. The treatment referred to was natural progesterone, which for more than 25 years has been hailed by Dr. Katharina Dalton as *the* cure for severe premenstrual syndrome. Dalton believes that PMS is a biological, hormonally based disorder which results from a relative deficiency of progesterone during the premenstrual phase. This deficiency, according to Dalton, creates a chemical (hormonal) imbalance which affects both the body and the mind.

The use of premenstrual syndrome as a mitigating circumstance in sentencing in criminal proceedings set a precedent in British courts and generated widespread discussion and controversy. The merits of the decisions were argued in editorials both in medical journals as well as in newspapers in Great Britain and elsewhere around the world (Gonzalez, 1981; *Lancet,* 1981; *South African Medical Journal,* 1981; *New York Times,* 1982).

The impact on the lay public, however, may be inferred from the large number of articles which have appeared in the past year or two in popular magazines. In the majority of these articles, both PMS and dysmenorrhea are discussed, with an emphasis on the argument that both "ailments" are physiologically based and are responsive to appropriate physiological treatment. In the case of dysmenorrhea, most writers cite the antiprostaglandin research, usually referring to Budoff's book. With respect to PMS, the arguments are less clear-cut, although Dalton's work is more often than not the focus of the piece.

The range of readership reached through these writings is impressive. A review of the recent periodical literature revealed articles in newsmagazines such as *Time* (Toufexis et al., 1981), *Newsweek* (Clark & Shapiro, 1981) and the *New York Times Magazine* (Henig, 1982), periodicals of general interest such as *People* (1982), and magazines for special interest groups (e.g., *Jet* 1981; Shangold, in *Runners World,* 1982). In addition, most of the major women's magazines have devoted space to discussions of PMS and dysmenorrhea (e.g., Agardy & Lancel in *Mademoiselle,* 1982; Brody, in *Ladies Home Journal,* 1981; Cohen, in *Mademoiselle,* 1981; Dwyer, in *Redbook,* 1980; Editorial in *Glamour,* 1981; O'Roark, in *McCall's,* 1981; and Weber & Holt, in *Vogue,* 1981).

With respect to their coverage of dysmenorrhea, most of these articles include valid information and provide a service to the readership. With respect to PMS, however, many authors present a rather distorted view. For one thing, there is a tendency on the part of some writers to lump together dysmenorrhea and PMS in proclaiming in a seemingly definitive fashion that for both problems there is a known physiological basis and a known and accepted physiological treatment. In most cases, even if they don't discuss it directly, the writers apparently accept Dalton's argument about both the basis (progesterone deficiency) and the treatment (administration of natural progesterone) of PMS. (*Note:* A notable exception to this trend is the well-balanced, carefully researched article by Henig, 1982).

It is important to recognize that although Dr. Dalton's opinions have been widely disseminated, truth in science can not ultimately be determined on the basis of popular beliefs. The exposure Dalton's work is currently receiving may very well be shaping public opinion. The fact remains, however, that there is little valid scientific evidence to support her claims for the effectiveness of natural progesterone. As was indicated in the Treatment section of this paper and in the thorough reviews of the Treatment literature referenced there, *no* treatment currently available can be cited as unconditionally suitable for sufferers of premenstrual syndrome.

The controversy over the relative effectiveness of progesterone pervades the scientific community as well, especially in Great Britain. The works of Dalton (1977), Sampson (1979), and O'Brien et al. (1980) have stimulated a lively debate as evidenced by letters to the *British Medical Journal* (e.g., Clare, 1980; Dalton, 1980a; 1980b; Martin & Downey, 1980; O'Brien, 1980; Sampson, 1980); to the *British Journal of Psychiatry* (e.g., Clare, 1981; Dalton, 1980), and editorials and letters in the *Lancet* (e.g., d'Orban, 1981; Editorial, 1981).

In both the scientific and the popular literature, one of the central issues tends to get lost, namely, that the effectiveness of any treatment must be evaluated in a context which includes both the meaning of the symptoms to the subject and the way she defines her participation in a treatment trial. Many women suffer from premenstrual problems for years, unable to convince physicians or other caregivers to take their complaints seriously. For many of these women, a treatment trial represents the first time anyone has really paid attention to the premenstrual difficulties. Thus, the potential "placebo" effect resulting from reassurance that she is not "crazy," that PMS is worthy of medical attention, etc., must be considered in any treatment study. And this is why, in the absence of such consideration, one must be somewhat skeptical of claims for any treatment modality which has not been shown repeatedly to be significantly superior to "placebo." It is this issue which needs to be communicated more effectively in the popular literature on PMS.

As both Dennerstein (1981) and Sampson (1981b) have pointed out, it is crucial that researchers and clinicians recognize the importance to PMS subjects and/or patients of having their complaints taken seriously by the health care provider. This advice extends to a recognition that PMS in its severe form is a problem not only for the individual woman, but for her family, as well.

REFERENCE NOTES

1. Alplanalp, J.M. Severe premenstrual syndrome: evaluation and assessment. Paper presented at annual meeting of American Society of Psychosomatic Obstetrics and Gynecology, Philadelphia, PA, March 1981.

2. Abplanalp, J.M. The severity of "severe" premenstrual tension syndrome. Paper presented at meeting of American College of Neuropsychopharmacology, San Diego, CA, December, 1981.

3. Haskett, R.F., & Abplanalp, J.M. Premenstrual tension syndrome: diagnostic criteria and the selection of research subjects. Submitted for publication, 1982.

4. Steiner, M., Haskett, R.F., Osmun, J., Rubin, R.T., & Carroll, B.J. Premenstrual tension syndrome—psychoendocrine evaluation and treatment outcome. Paper presented at American Psychosomatic Society, Annual Meeting, Dallas, TX, March, 1979.

REFERENCES

Abplanalp, J.M., Hasket, R.F., & Rose, R.M. The premenstrual syndrome. *Psychiatric Clinics of North America*, 1980, *3*, 327-347.

Abraham, G. The premenstrual tension syndromes. In: L.K. McNale (Ed.) *Contemporary obstetric and gynecologic nursing*. New York: C.V. Mosby, 1980, 170-184.

Abraham, G.E., & Lubran, M.M. Serum and red cell magnesium levels in patients with premenstrual tension. *American Journal of Clinical Nutrition*, 1981, *34*, 2364-2366.

Adamopoulos, D.A., Loraine, J.A., Lunn, S.F., Coppen, A.J., & Daly, R.J. Endocrine profiles in premenstrual tension. *Clinical Endocrinology*, 1972, *1*, 283-292.

Agardy, M., & Lancel, K. Can you exercise menstrual troubles away? *Mademoiselle*, 1982, *88*, 52.

Andersch, B., Hahn, L., Anderson, M., & Isaksson, B. Body water and weight in patients with premenstrual tension. *British Journal of Obstetrics and Gynecology*, 1978a, *85*, 546-550.

Andersch, B., Hahn, L., Wendestam, C., Ohman, R., & Abrahamsson, L. Treatment of premenstrual tension syndrome with bromocriptine. *Acta Endocrinologica Supplement 216*, 1978b, *88*, 165-174.

Andersch, B., Abrahamsson, L., Wendestam, C., Ohman, R., & Hahn, L. Hormone profile in premenstrual tension: Effects of bromocriptine and diuretics. *Clinical Endocrinology*, 1979, *11*, 657-664.

Andersen, A.N., Larsen, J.F., Streenstrup, O.R., Svendstrup, B., & Nielson, J. Effect of bromocriptine on the premenstrual syndrome: A double-blind clinical trial. *British Journal of Obstetrics and Gynecology*, 1977, *84*, 370-374.

Backstrom, T., & Carstensen, H. Estrogen and progesterone in plasma in relation to premenstrual tension. *Journal of Steroid Biochemistry*, 1974, *5*, 257-260.

Backstrom, T., & Mattson, B. Correlation in symptoms in premenstrual tension to estrogen and progesterone concentrations in blood plasma. *Neuropsychobiology*, 1975, *1*, 80-86.

Backstrom, T. Wide, L., Sodergard, R., & Carstensen, H. FSH, LH TeBG—capacity, estrogen and progesterone in women with premenstrual tension during the luteal phase. *Journal of Steroid Biochemistry*, 1976, *7*, 473-476.

Backstrom, T., Boyle, H., & Baird, D.T. Persistence of symptoms in premenstrual tension in hysterectimized women. *British Journal of Obstetrics and Gynecology*, 1981, *88*, 530-536.

Backstrom, T., & Aakvaag, A. Plasma prolactin and testosterone during the luteal phase in women with premenstrual tension syndrome. *Psychoneuroendocrinologica*, 1981, *6*, (3), 245-251.

Benedek-Jaszmann, L.J., & Hearn-Sturtevant, M.D. Premenstrual tension and functional infertility. Aetiology and treatment. *Lancet*, 1976, *1*, 1095-1098.

Brody, J. Menstrual problems. Lifting "the curse" at last. *Ladies Home Journal*, 1981, *98*, 44.

Budoff, P. *No more menstrual cramps, and other good news*. New York: Putnam, 1980.

Carroll, B.J., & Steiner, M. The psychobiology of premenstrual dysphoria: The role of prolactin. *Psychoneuroendocrinologica*, 1978, *3*, 171-180.

Clare, A.W. The treatment of premenstrual symptoms. *Brittish Journal of Psychiatry*, 1979, *135*, 576-579.

Clare, A.W. Progesterone, fluid and electrolytes in premenstrual syndrome (Letter). *British Medical Journal*, 1980, *281*, 810-811.

Clare, A.W. Premenstrual syndrome (Letter). *British Journal of Psychiatry*, 1981, *138*, 82-83.

Clare, A.W. Psychiatric aspects of premenstrual complaint. *Journal of Psychosomatic Obstetrics and Gynecology*, 1982, *1*, 22-31.

Clark, M., & Shapiro, D. Monthly syndrome. *Newsweek*, 1981, *97*, 74.

Cohen, S.S. Premenstrual syndrome. *Mademoiselle*, 1981, *87*, 57-58.

Crime and premenstrual tension (Editorial). *South African Medical Journal*, 1981, *60*, 877.

Culberg, J. Mood changes and menstrual symptoms with different gestagen/estrogen combinations. *Acta Psychiatrica Scandinavica*, 1972, Suppl. 236.

Dalton, K. *The premenstrual syndrome*. London: Heinemann Medical, 1964.

Dalton, K. *The premenstrual syndrome and progesterone therapy*. London: Heinemann Medical, 1977.

Dalton, K. Progesterone, fluid and electrolytes in premenstrual syndrome (Letter). *British Medical Journal*, 1980a, *281*, 61.

Dalton, K. Progesterone, fluid and electrolytes in premenstrual syndrome (Letter). *British Medical Journal*, 1980b, *281*, 1008-1009.

Dennerstein, L. Discussion. In: P.A. vanKeep & W.H. Utian (Eds) *The premenstrual syndrome*. Lancaster, England: MTP Press, Ltd., 1981.

d'Orban, P.T. Premenstrual syndrome: A disease of the mind? (Letter). *Lancet*, 1981, *2*, 1413.

Dwyer, J. Menstruation and food cravings (interview). *Redbook*, 1980, *155*, 46.

Editorial. *New York Times*, 1982, *18*, 1.

Elsner, C.W., Buster, J.E., Schindler, R.A., Nessim, S.A., & Abraham, G.E. Bromocriptine in the treatment of premenstrual tension syndrome. *Obstetrics and Gynecology*, 1980, *56*, 723-726.

Endicott, J., Halbreich, U., Schacht, S., & Nee, J. Premenstrual changes and affective disorders. *Psychosomatic Medicine*, 1981, *43*, 519-530.

Frank, R.T. The hormonal causes of premenstrual tension. *Archives of Neurology and Psychiatry*, 1931, *26*, 1053-1057.

Ghose, K., & Coppen, A. Bromocriptine and premenstrual syndrome: Controlled study. *British Medical Journal*, 1977, *209*, 147-148.

Glamour editorial (Report on America's attitudes toward menstruation). *Glamour*, 1981, *79*, 82.

Gonzalez, E.R. Premenstrual syndrome: An ancient woe deserving of modern scrutiny (News). *Journal of the American Medical Association*, 1981, *245*, 1393-1396.

Graham, J.J., Harding, P.E., Wise, P.H., & Berriman, H. Prolactin suppression in the treatment of premenstrual syndrome. *The Medical Journal of Australia, Special Supplement*, 1978, 18-20.

Halbreich, U., Assael, M., Ben-David, & Borstein, R. Serum prolactin in women with premenstrual syndrome. *Lancet*, 1976, *2*, 654-56.

Halbreich, U., & Endicott, J. Classification of premenstrual syndromes. In: R. Friedman (Ed.) *Behavior and the menstrual cycle*. New York: Marcel Dekker, 1982.

Halbreich, U., Endicott, J., Schacht, S., & Nee, J. Premenstrual assessment form: A new procedure to reflect the diversity of premenstrual changes. *Acta Psychiatrica Scandinavica*, 1982, *65*, 46-65.

Haskett, R.F., Steiner, M., Osman, J.N., & Carroll, B.J. Severe premenstrual tension: Delineation of the syndrome. *Biological Psychiatry*, 1980, *15*, 121-139.

Henig, R.M. Dispelling menstrual myths. *New York Times Magazine*, 1982, p. 64.

Horrobin, D.F. Premenstrual syndrome and pregnancy toxemia. In: *Prolactin: Physiology and clinical significance*. Lancaster, Eng: MTP Press, 1973, 115-120.

"In England two killers go free on grounds they were victims of premenstrual tension." *People*, 1982, *17*, 94.

Martin, A.J., & Downey, L.J. Progesterone, fluid and electrolytes in premenstrual syndrome. (Letter). *British Medical Journal*, 1980, *281*, 562-563.

Moos, R.H., & Leiderman, D.B. Toward a conceptualization of menstrual symptom types. *Journal of Psychosomatic Research*, 1978, *22*, 31-40.

O'Brien, P.M.S., Selby, C., & Symonds, E.M. Progesterone, fluid and electrolytes in premenstrual syndrome. *British Medical Journal*, 1980, *280*, 1161-1163.

O'Brien, P.M.S. Progesterone, fluid, and electrolytes (Letter). *British Medical Journal*, 1980, *281*, 563.

O'Roark, M.A. Your once-a-month mood changes (premenstrual tension). *McCall's*, 1981, *108*, 12+.

Parlee, M.B. The premenstrual syndrome. *Psychological Bulletin*, 1973, *80*, 454-465.

Premenstrual syndrome (Editorial). *Lancet*, 1981, *2*, 1393-1394.

Reid, R.L., & Yen, S.S.C. Premenstrual syndrome. *American Journal of Obstetrics and Gynecology*, 1981, *139*, 85-104.

Ruble, D.N., & Brooks-Gunn, J. Menstrual symptoms: A social cognition analysis. *Journal of Behavioral Medicine*, 1979, *2*, 171-193.

Sampsom, G.A. Premenstrual syndrome: A double-blind controlled trial of progesterone and placebo. *British Journal of Psychiatry*, 1979, *135*, 209-215.

Sampson, G.A. Progesterone, fluid, and electrolytes in premenstrual syndrome (Letter). *British Medical Journal*, 1980, *281*, 227-228.

Sampson, G.A. An appraisal of the role of progesterone in the therapy of premenstrual syndrome. In: P.A. vanKeep & W.H. Utian (Eds.). *The premenstrual syndrome*. Lancaster, Eng: MTP Press, Ltd., 1981a, 51-69.

Sampson, G.A. Discussion. In: P.A. vanKeep & W.H. Utian, (Eds.) *The premenstrual syndrome*. Lancaster, Eng: MTP Press, Ltd., 1981b, p. 98.

Sampson, G.A., & Prescott, P. The assessment of the symptoms of premenstrual syndrome and their response to therapy. *British Journal of Psychiatry*, 1981, *138*, 399-495.

Shangold, M. Women's running. *Runners World*, 1982, *17*, 21.

Smith, S.L. Mood and the menstrual cycle. In: E. Sacher (Ed.) *Topics in psychoendocrinology*. New York: Grune & Stratton, 1975. 19-58.

Sommer, B. Stress and menstrual distress. *Journal of Human Stress*, 1978, *4*, 1-10, 41-47.

Steiner, M., & Carroll, B.J. The psychobiology of premenstrual dysphoria: Review of theories and treatments. *Psychoneuroendocrinologica*, 1977, *2*, 321-335.

Tonks, C.M. Premenstrual tension. *British Journal of Psychiatry, Special Publication #9*, 1975, 399-408.

Toufexis, A. Coping with Eve's curse. *Time*, 1981, *118*, 59.

Weber, M., & Holt, L.H. Inner information: Menstruation. *Vogue*, 1981, *171*, 344-345.

"Women may be abusive due to premenstrual stress." *Jet*, 1981, *60*, 23.

The Relationship between Psychopathology and the Menstrual Cycle

Anthony W. Clare, MD

ABSTRACT. Higher rates of mental ill-health, particularly mood disorder, have been reported in women compared to men and this discrepancy has been attributed to underlying biological changes associated with the menstrual cycle. The literature relating to psychiatric ill-health and the premenstrual syndrome is, accordingly, critically evaluated and the evidence favouring a causal role for menstrual cycle changes in the genesis of such ill-health is briefly reviewed. A simple model of causation attributing psychiatric-ill-health to hormonal variation in the menstrual cycle is eschewed in favour of a multifactorial model which assumes an interaction between hormonal and hormonally-related changes in the premenstruum, basic personality and social dissatisfactions, adverse life circumstances, and interpersonal stresses.

As has been pointed out in a recent and thorough review of the subject, there is a persistent reporting of excess psychiatric morbidity in women compared with men for which no single explanation appears sufficient (Briscoe, 1982). Given that there are almost certainly psychological and social factors contributing to the reported excess of female psychiatric morbidity, is there any evidence of a biological contribution and for an association between such a contribution and the biological changes associated with the menstrual cycle (Briscoe, 1982; Gove & Tudor, 1973; Nathanson, 1975)? Despite a considerable literature devoted to the premenstrual syndrome (Smith, 1975; Abplanalp et al., 1980; Clare, in press), the precise relationship between psychiatric morbidity and premenstrual complaint has been poorly studied and remains shadowy.

In examining such literature as is available and such studies as have been undertaken, it is best if psychiatric disorders are somewhat arbitrarily broken down into psychotic illnesses, neurotic illnesses, and personality disorders. The distinction between these classes, and particularly the last two, is necessarily arbitrary but it is necessary for the sake of clarity.

PREMENSTRUAL SYMPTOMS AND PSYCHOTIC ILLNESS

There is a well-documented array of studies which support the view that many recurrent psychotic illnesses flare up in the premenstrual phase of afflicted women more often than would be expected by chance (Smith, 1975). Analysis of female admissions to psychiatric hospitals and units in relation to phase of cycle at the time of admission has shown a similar pattern. Dalton (1959) studied 276 mental hospital admissions and found distinct peaks at the premenstrual, menstrual and ovulatory phases. Janowsky and his colleagues (1969) found that 27 of 44 general hospital psychiatric admissions had occurred between five days before and five days after the onset of the menses. Of 435 admissions to a Danish mental hospital, 183 (42%) concerned women in the premenstrual phase at the time of admission (Kramp, 1968). One hundred forty-six women had "a well-characterized premenstrual syndrome." Another study involving 271 patients in state mental hospitals claimed that 216 (79%) had "premenstrual tension" (Torghele, 1957) while a Japanese cohort of patients diagnosed as suffering from "periodic psychosis" showed a highly significant correlation between acute recurrence and the luteal phase of the cycle (Wakoh et al., 1960).

More recently, a definitely increased prevalence of premenstrual mood change has been reported in women with primary affective disorder compared with women diagnosed as suffering from anxiety or hysteria (Kashiwagi et al., 1976). The criteria used by this team of researchers included psychological and physical symptoms commonly reported premenstrually and the psychiatric diagnosis of affective disorder was that established by Feighner and his colleagues (Feighner et al., 1972). However, the groups studied was a somewhat arbitrary sample in that the women, 75% of whom were black, had all been originally referred to a neurology clinic for functional headache. A better designed study compared women with previously diagnosed affective illness with a control group and found no difference with respect to somatic symptoms complained of around menstruation (Diamond et al., 1976). So-called dysphoria in relation to the menstrual cycle showed only a slight trend toward increased reporting by the affective group. There was a tendency for women to be hospitalised for depression during the late premenstrual phase of the cycle. The authors of this study interpreted their findings as suggesting that women predisposed to affective disorders, but not suffering from a current episode, experience menstruation in much the same way as normal women do. On the other hand, patients in the middle of an affective episode may experience a premenstrual exacerbation of their current symptoms so that hospital admission is often precipitated at that time. To date, this does appear to be the explanation best supported by the available literature concerning the association between psychosis and premenstrual symptomatology.

PREMENSTRUAL SYMPTOMS AND NEUROTIC ILLNESS

Whereas there is an extensive literature devoted to the association between psychotic illness and premenstrual symptomatology, there are only a handful of studies in the literature concerned with the possible link between neurosis and the syndrome. Rees studied patients attending a psychiatric outpatient department, a psychosomatic and allergy clinic, and a sample of "normal" women, and reported a significant association between severe premenstrual tension syndrome and neurosis (Rees, 1953). However, the association was not absolute and Rees observed that "premenstrual tension can exist in women with little or no evidence of instability in personality adjustment or of neurosis or of predisposition to neurosis" and conversely that "many women with severe neurosis do not suffer from premenstrual tension." Rees argued that a history of childhood neurosis, personality instability, and clinical abnormality acted as intervening variables explaining the link between severe neurosis and premenstrual tension.

Coppen's study of 151 psychiatric patients included 49 with a diagnosis of "neurosis" (Coppen, 1965). Compared with controls, the neurotic patients complained more frequently of irritability, depression, and pain, but it is not absolutely clear from the published study whether these symptoms were more commonly reported premenstrually. Coppen indicated that for the group of psychiatric patients as a whole, irritability, depression, headaches, and swelling were more commonly complained of premenstrually whereas pain was a phenomenon associated with menstruation. But elsewhere in the paper he reveals that neurotic patients complained significantly more of irritability, depression, and headaches at other times in the menstrual cycle compared with controls.

The shortcomings of Coppen's studies are similar to those of Rees's work. There is no standardized definition of what constitutes neurosis nor are details provided of how clinical information leading to a diagnosis of psychiatric ill-health was made. There was confusion between menstrual and premenstrual symptoms which has rather important implications for the findings, given that elsewhere it has been claimed that menstrual pain is not associated with neurotic symptomatology whereas premenstrual pain is (Kessel & Coppen, 1963). The only somatic symptoms inquired about were "swelling" and "headaches" and the only psychological symptoms were "irritability" and "depression, anxiety and nervous tension." Nevertheless, Coppen's findings suggest that in this study, as in the study by Diamond and her colleagues on the relationship between affective disorder and premenstrual complaints, the patients differed from the controls only in terms of their experience of psychological symptoms premenstrually, there being no difference in experience of physical symptoms premenstrually (Diamond et al., 1976). The controls used by Coppen in his study were drawn from a community survey and while matched with patients for age and parity they were not matched for social class. The sample included in-patients and out-patients and no attempt was made to establish whether admission status affected the significance of the findings. Finally, the lack of any explicit definition of neurosis makes it difficult to rule out the possibility of contamination between the manner whereby it was assessed and the way in which the presence or absence of premenstrual symptoms was established.

Recently, a study aimed at clarifying the relationship between premenstrual complaint and psychiatric ill-health has been undertaken in women attending general practitioners in Britain (Clare, 1977; Clare, Note 1; Clare, in press). To screen 521 women attending 25 general practitioners, use was made of a modifed version of the Menstrual Distress Questionnaire (Moos, 1968) and the General Health Questionnaire (Goldberg, 1972), an instrument specifically designed and validated as a screening tool to detect psychiatrically ill individuals in the general population. A subsample of women, drawn by virtue of the nature of their responses on the two questionnaires, was interviewed by means of a standardized, semi-structured psychiatric interview (Goldberg et al., 1970). A highly significant association between premenstrual complaint and psychiatric ill-health was found. Psychiatrically ill premenstrual complainers differed from psychiatrically healthy complainers in that they reported significantly more behavioural and psychological symptoms premenstrually. The two groups did not differ significantly with respect to their tendency to complain of physical symptoms premenstrually. Psychiatrically ill premenstrual complainers did complain of a more severe form of premenstrual disorder, but this was true only with respect to psychological symptoms such as depression, irritability, and tension, and to a lesser extent behavioural disturbances such as loss of efficiency and the avoidance of social activities. Psychiatrically ill premenstrual complainers did not complain of a more severe experience of physical symptoms, such as breast tenderness, cramps, headache, backache, or swelling, than that complained of by psychiatrically healthy premenstrual complainers.

The women in this study were also assessed in terms of their social functioning, as assessed by a standardized, semi-structured schedule (Clare & Cairns, 1978). Although there was no significant association between premenstrual complaint and overall social maladjustment, there was a positive but not significant trend for disturbances in marital function to be associated with premenstrual complaint that was independent of psychiatric status.

PREMENSTRUAL SYMPTOMS
AND PERSONALITY DISTURBANCES

An association between deficiencies in personality growth and structure and premenstrual complaint has long been suggested. Morton claimed that premenstrual tension was commonest in emotionally unstable women (Morton, 1950), and Coppen and Kessel found that women with severe premenstrual irritability or depression had significantly higher scores on the Maudsley Personality Inventory Scale (MPIS) than did unaffected women (Coppen & Kessel, 1963). Even when the MPIS was modified to remove items that might have been influenced by menstrual symptoms, such a finding persisted. Subjects with irregular periods also had high neuroticism scores, whereas subjects with dysmenorrhoea did not.

Several other studies indicate a possible relationship between menstrual or premenstrual complaints on the one hand and a general "neurotic" or "psychosomatic complaining" tendency on the other

(Smith, 1975). These studies include a poorly designed question-naire (Levitt & Lubin, 1967) and a claim by Kramp (1968) that in "mental patients" the premenstrual syndrome is more frequently found in persons who had neurotic symptoms in childhood.

Some studies, mainly psychoanalytical in orientation, have fo-cused on the extent to which a woman's psychological response to the physiological changes associated with the menstrual cycle might be shaped or modified by cultural practices that attach value to men-struation and to femininity (Thompson, 1950; Shainess, 1961; Paige, 1971). Shainess, for example, sent questionnaires to more than a hundred women, including her own analytic patients, and concluded, at least to her own satisfaction, that most of the reported menstrual problems related to traumatic or badly handled ex-periences of the menarche (Shainess, 1961). Helene Deutsch stressed the importance of the mother-daughter relationship in determining subsequent attitudes toward the menses and associated symptomatology (Deutsch, 1944); others, following a similar line of thought, have emphasized the rejection of the feminine role, guilt over sexual temptation, and diminished comfort in the mature feminine role (Menninger, 1939; Fortin et al., 1958; Paulson, 1961). Hain and his colleagues claimed an association between menstrual irregularity and premenstrual symptoms and that MMPI scores indicating personality abnormalities were associated with menstrual irregularity (Hain et al., 1970). Factor analysis in this study produced six factors, one of which, "normal personality," correlated negatively with the factors "premenstrual tension" and "premenstrual headache" and positively with the factor "freedom from menstrual symptoms." In another study, women described as apprehensive, cautious, conventional, stable, and unemotional tend-ed to report little peri-menstrual symptomatology, whereas women described as shy, self-doubting, eager to seek help, and tending to behave in a self-defeating way tended to report more such symp-tomatology (Gough, 1975).

Many of the above studies, however, have profound flaws in design, sampling, and instruments of measurement, and show a sturdy resistance to considering alternative explanations for their findings. A more recent study, which suffers from a number of flaws as well (the sample is selected in a somewhat nondescript fashion, for instance), nonetheless represents a more thorough at-tempt to clarify the relationship between psychological factors and premenstrual symptomatology (Taylor, 1979). Using the Eysenck

Personality Inventory, Cattell's 16 Personality Factor Questionnaire (16PF), and a daily symptom rating scale made up of a reasonable cross section of the more common premenstrual symptoms, the author found a strong association between neuroticism and high levels of premenstrual symptoms. Women positive with respect to at least two of the four criteria of troublesome premenstrual symptoms differed significantly from women positive for only one or none of these criteria.

The results suggested a personality profile of high premenstrual complaint scorers with the following characteristics: emotionally unstable, suspicious, unpretentious, guilt-prone, apprehensive, self-conflicted, tense, and frustrated. Taylor speculated that the physiological changes associated with menstruation are associated with mild changes in behaviour and mood, changes which occur in the great majority of women. At the extremes of the normal range, these changes may be of a sufficient magnitude to be unpleasant. Some women will be particularly sensitive to menstrual phenomena, possibly because of psychological and social attitudes toward menstruation and associated taboos. Some women may be more sensitive to minor physiological changes and some at least of these women may have particularly low thresholds for detecting such stimuli. The physiological changes, therefore, may be within normal limits but their subjective appreciation of these changes will be magnified by their sensitization. Such women may report high symptom ratings and may well account for most of the subjects with high ratings, although most will not seek treatment for these symptoms. Finally, some women who report severe symptoms and do seek treatment on that account are, in Taylor's view, probably similar to neurotic patients and can be expected to score high on tests on which neurotic patients also score high.

IMPLICATIONS FOR MANAGEMENT

Clinical experience suggests that whereas so-called "pure" PMT, i.e., uncontaminated by psychosocial factors, responds usually quite well to one or other of the physical treatments currently available and endorsed as suitable for this condition (Clare, 1979), the form of the condition associated with psychosocial difficulties and psychiatric ill-health responds poorly unless such treatments are accompanied by interventions aimed at identifying and possibly easing the associated difficulties. But a word of caution is required both for patients and their therapists. Many women feel threatened by any suggestion that their premenstrual disturbances might in any way be related to or exacerbated by associated psychological or interpersonal difficulties. Many spouses appear to feel even more threatened. Women feel threatened because they tend to believe that such an explanation suggests that they are fabricating their premenstrual complaints and have some investment in retaining the complaints in order to prove that they are "real." Many spouses feel threatened because any suggestion that their wives' hormonal oddities might in some way be less important than, for example, the marital relationship, brings them out of the shadows into the limelight in a manner which alters their role from being those sympathetic confidantes encouraging their wives to rectify their abnormal reproductive system to being potential causal agents in their own right.

The view that certain gynaecological symptoms such as pelvic pain are either "real" or "imaginary" and that psychosocial factors can only be involved in "imaginary" symptoms is widespread amongst both patients and doctors according to Beard and his obstetrical colleagues at St. Mary's in London (Pearce et al., 1982). It is, however, a distinction which is untenable in view of considerable recent research on pain (Weisenberg, 1980) and on the role of psychological factors in a wide variety of physical conditions from appendicitis (Creed, 1981) to cardiovascular disease (Friedman et al., 1975). In clarifying and establishing the association between psychiatric ill-health and premenstrual complaint in women one runs the risk of actually enhancing the tendency of some physicians to dismiss women who complain of premenstrual tension as "neurotic" and of attributing the occurrence of symptoms to the operation of such alleged neurotic factors as a refusal to accept feminine status or a peculiar and particular manifestation of hypochondriasis! For such reasons, many female commentators in this area (Delaney et al., 1977; Weidegar, 1978) view with trepidation mixed with hostility any argument which appears to suggest that premenstrual complaint or dysmenorrhoea is "all in the mind."

In fact, however, the identification of co-existing psychosocial difficulties exacerbating or even causally contributing to premenstrual symptoms or even assuming a greater significance than any such symptoms, requires that the physician take a broader approach to the patient than that involving the prescription of a physical treatment. As Pearce and her colleagues have demonstrated in the management of the common gynaecological problem pelvic pain (Pearce et al., 1982), simple, non-directive exploratory counselling with or without group support and or relaxation can be particularly helpful. Clinical experience suggests that for many a woman clarification of the extent to which marital and/or other personal difficulties account for and contribute to the dismal and depressing way she feels, far from depressing and discouraging her further, can often help improve her own self-esteem. Attributing each and every symptom of distress to an alleged defect in a woman's hormonal system can in its own way be as dispiriting as blaming it all on her nerves, and can lead to "the discounting of situational factors and an emphasis on biology" (Koeske & Koeske, 1975).

Simply to assume that any woman who complains of premenstrual symptoms or dysmenorrhoea must be "neurotic" ignores the fact that a small but significant number of women do manifest such symptoms in a consistent and convincing manner suggestive of an underlying biological disturbance albeit one which hitherto remains undetected. Likewise, simply to assume that any and every dissatisfaction and discomfort experienced by a woman during her active reproductive life is the consequence of her menstrual cycle envisages women as the prisoners and products of their cyclical functions. Both positions have a long historical tradition. The first was held with particular conviction by psychiatrists towards the turn of the century and has been maintained particularly by psychoanalysts, one of whom, the influential Karen Horney, confidently attributed premenstrual symptoms to repressed sexual desire and power (Horney, 1931). The second was much prized by gynaecologists, also at the turn of the century, many of whom tended to regard the whole state of being a woman as a major health hazard in its own right! Such a view was most eloquently expressed by the President of the American Gynaecological Society when in 1900 he observed:

> Many a young life is battered and forever crippled in the breakers of puberty; if it crosses these unharmed and is not dashed to pieces on the rock of childbirth, it may still ground on the ever-recurring shallows of menstruation, and lastly, upon the final bar of the menopause ere protection is found in the unruffled waters of the harbor beyond the reach of sexual storms. (Englemann, 1900)

Today, there is a change of a similar polarization concerning the underlying nature of conditions such as dysmenorrhoea and premenstrual tension occurring. However, such evidence as is available suggests that a multifactorial model of causation and treatment may well be more appropriate. Such an approach assumes on interaction between hormonal and hormonally related changes in the premenstruum, the basic personality, including perhaps the woman's basic attitude to and threshold for pain and other discomforts, and social dissatisfactions, adverse life circumstances, and interpersonal stresses.

REFERENCE NOTE

1. Clare, A. W. Psychiatric and social aspects of premenstrual complaint. M.D. Thesis. National University of Ireland, University College Dublin, 1981.

REFERENCES

Abplanalp, J.M., Haskett, R.F., & Rose, R.M. The premenstrual syndrome. *Psychiatric Clinics of North America*, 1980, *3*, 327-347.

Briscoe, M.E. Subjective measures of well-being; differences in the perception of health and social problems. *British Journal of Social Work*, 1982, *12*(2), 137-147.

Clare, A.W., & Cairns, V.E. Design, development and use of a standardised interview to assess social maladjustment and dysfunction in community studies. *Psychological Medicine*, 1978, *8*, 589-604.

Clare, A.W. Psychological problems of women complaining of premenstrual symptoms. *Current Medical Research & Opinion*, 1977, *4*(4), 23-28.

Clare, A.W. The treatment of premenstrual symptoms. *British Journal of Psychiatry*, 1979, *135*, 576-579.

Clare, A.W. Psychiatric and social aspects of premenstrual complaint. *Psychological Medicine*, in press.

Coppen, A. The prevalence of menstrual disorders in psychiatric patients. *British Journal of Psychiatry*, 1965, *111*, 155-167.

Creed, R. Life events and appendicectomy. *Lancet*, 1981, *1*, 1381-1385.

Dalton, K. Menstruation and acute psychiatric illness. *British Medical Journal*, 1959, *1*, 148.

Delaney, J., Lufton, M.J., & Toth, E. *The curse: A cultural history of menstruation.* New York: New American Library, 1977.

Deutsch, H. *The psychology of women.* New York: Grune & Stratton, 1944.

Diamond, S.B., Rubenstein, A.A., Dunner, D.I., et al. Menstrual problems in women with primary affective illness. *Comprehensive Psychiatry*, 1976, *17*, 541.

Engelmann, G.E. The American girl of today: Modern education and functional health. Quoted in Smith-Rosenberg, C. & Rosenberg, C. The female animal: Medical and biological views of woman and her role in the 19th century America. *Journal of American History*, 1973, *60*, 336-337.

Feighner, J.R., Robins, E., Guze, S.B. et al. Diagnositc criteria for use in psychiatric research. *Archives of General Psychiatry*, 1972, *26*, 57.

Fortin, J.N., Wittilower, E.D., & Kalz, F. Psychosomatic approach to premenstrual tension syndrome: A preliminary report. *Canadian Medical Association Journal*, 1958, *79*, 978-981.

Friedman, M., Byers, B., Diamant, J., & Rosenhan, R.H. Plasma catecholamine response of coronary-prone subjects (type A) to a specific challenge. *Metabolism*, 1975, *24*, 205-210.

Goldberg, D. *The detection of psychiatric illness by questionnaire*. Maudsley Monograph No. 21. London: Oxford University Press, 1972.

Goldberg, D.P., Cooper, B., Eastwood, M.R., Kedward, H.P., & Shepherd, M. A standardized psychiatric interview for use in community surveys. *British Journal of Preventive Social Medicine*, 1970, *24*, 118-123.

Gough, H.G. Personality factors related to reported severity of menstrual disress. *Journal of Abnormal Psychology*, 1975, *84* (1), 59-65.

Gove, W.R., & Tudor, J.F. Adult sex roles and mental illness. *American Journal of Sociology*, 1973, *78*, 812-835.

Hain, J.D., Linton, P.H., Ebor, H.W., & Chapman, M.M. Menstrual irregularity, symptoms and personality. *Journal of Psychosomatic Research*, 1970, *14*, 81-87.

Horney, K. Die Premenstruelle Verstimmungen. *Feminine Psychology*. New York: Norton, 1967.

Janowsky, D.S., Gorney, R., Castelnuovo-Tedesco, P. et al. Premenstrual-menstrual neurosis in psychiatric hospital admission notes. *American Journal of Obstetrics & Gynaecology*, 1969, *103*, 189.

Kashiwagi, T., McClure, Jr. J.N., & Wetzel, R.D. Premenstrual affective syndrome and psychiatric disorder. *Diseases of the Nervous System*, 1976, *37*, 116.

Kessel, N., & Coppen, A. Menstruation and personality. *British Journal of Psychiatry*, 1963, *109*, 711-721.

Koeske, R.K., & Koeske, G.F. An attributional approach to moods and the menstrual cycle. *Journal of Personality & Social Psychology*, 1975, *31*, 473.

Kramp, J.L. Studies on the premenstrual syndrome in relation to psychiatry. *Acta Psychiatrica Scandinavica (Suppl.)* 1968, *203*, 261.

Levitt, E.E., & Lubin, B. Some personality factors associated with menstrual complaints and menstrual attitudes. *Journal of Psychosomatic Research*, 1967, *11*, 267-270.

Menninger K.A. Somatic correlations with the unconscious repudiation of femininity in women. *Journal of Nervous and Mental Disease*, 1939, *89*, 514-527.

Moos, R.H. The development of a menstrual distress questionnaire. *Psychosomatic Medicine*, 1968, *30*, 863-867.

Morton, J.H. Premenstrual tension. *American Journal of Obstetrics and Gynecology*, 1950, *60*, 343-352.

Nathanson, C.A. Illness and the feminine role: A theoretical review. *Social Science & Medicine*, 1975, *9*, 57-62.

Paulson, M.J. Psychological concomitants of premenstrual tension. *American Journal of Obstetrics and Gynecology*, 1961, *81*, 733-738.

Paige, K. Effects of oral contraceptives on affective fluctuations associated with the menstrual cycle. *Psychosomatic Medicine*, 1971, *33*, 515-537.

Pearce, S., Knight, C., & Beard, R.W. Pelvic pain: A common gynaecological problem. *Journal of Psychosomatic Obstetrics & Gynaecology*, 1982, *1*, 12-17.

Rees, I. Psychosomatic aspects of the premenstrual syndrome. *Journal of Mental Science*, 1953, *99*, 62-73.

Shainess, N. A re-evaluation of some aspects of femininity through a study of menstruation: A preliminary report. *Comprehensive Psychiatry*, 1961, *2*, 20-26.

Smith, S.L. Mood and the menstrual cycle. In E. J. Sacher (Ed.) *Topics in psychoendocrinology*. New York: Grune & Stratton, 1975.

Taylor, J.W. Psychological factors in the aetiology of premenstrual symptoms. *Australian and New Zealand Journal of Psychiatry*, 1979, *13*, 35-41.

Thompson, C. Some effects of the derogatory attitude toward female sexuality. *Psychiatry*, 1950, *13*, 349-354.

Torghele, J.R. Premenstrual tension in psychotic women. *Lancet*, 1957, *77*, 163-170.

Wakoh, T., Takedoshi, A., Yoshimoto, S. et al. Pathophysiological study of the periodic psychosis (atypical endogenous psychosis) with special reference to the comparison with chronic schizophrenia. *Mie Medical Journal*, 1960, *10*, 317.

Weideger, P. *Menstruation and menopause.* New York: Knopf, 1976.

Menopause:
The Closure of Menstrual Life

Ann M. Voda, RN, PhD
Mona Eliasson, PhD

ABSTRACT. This paper discusses questions frequently asked by menopausal women regarding body and affective changes associated with the menopause. Menopause as disease is contrasted with menopause as normal. Common menopausal changes and ways in which to deal with them are presented. Answers to some of the questions and concerns that women have cannot be found in the research done to date because of lack of unbiased research on the normalcy of menopause. Thus, this paper illustrates the need for woman-centered research to answer women-related phenomena.

Menopause is one of the most definitive landmarks of aging in women. It is a universal and normal development event for all women. Yet women can expect to live 30 or more years postmenopause and the commonly reported changes associated with menopause have only recently been the focus of serious research endeavors. Scant scientific data exist as to the nature of menopause as a transitional stage in women's development and more information is needed about the changes associated with the menopausal transition. The hot flash, for example, was virtually ignored as a subject of serious research until Molnar (1975) reported the experience of one subject. Only medical case studies were reported prior to Molnar's work and they merely supported the assumption of menopause as disease by the medical establishment.

Dr. Voda would like to acknowledge the financial assistance of the Health and Human Services, Health Resources Administration, Bureau of Health Manpower, Division of Nursing, through grant # R01 NU 00961, and appreciation to James Tucker for secretarial, technical, and editing assistance.

137

MENOPAUSE AS DISEASE

Despite the fact that little was and is known about the menopause, the hot flash, or other body changes, menopausal women have been widely and indiscriminately treated with estrogens. A noted San Francisco gynecologist summed up the attitude of the medical establishment when he said, "I think of the menopause as a deficiency disease, like diabetes . . . so I prescribe estrogen for virtually all menopausal women for an indefinite period" (MacPherson, 1981).

In current medical literature menopausal women are described as hypogonadal, castrates, or as estrogen deficient. Implicit in such labeling is a message that the totality of aging womanhood has been reduced to the level of the gonads. At menopause, then, a woman is not wholly a woman without functional gonads, nor is she a man.

What then is a menopausal woman? Unfortunately, the view taken by medical practitioners is that women are estrogen deficient! Such a definition is consistent with the menopause as disease concept which led to millions of women being placed on estrogen so as to prevent aging and uterine cancer. Unfortunately for many women, however, there was a high price to be paid for the indiscriminate use of estrogen and acceptance of the myth that all menopausal women are diseased. Specifically, in 1975 the first reports appeared in the *New England Journal of Medicine* that suggested a link between a reported increased incidence of uterine cancer in women and estrogen replacement therapy (Smith, Prentice, Thompson, & Herrman, 1975; Ziel & Finkle, 1975). In 1977, despite the 1975 reports, it was estimated that 4.1 million women in the United States were treated with estrogen replacement therapy (ERT). Also in 1977, the FDA warned women about the ERT-cancer association; and in 1979 an NIH Consensus Conference on ERT-Menopause concluded that ERT is risky, that women users should be fully informed regarding risks, and that alternatives to ERT are needed as well as research aimed at describing the natural history of menopause (NIH, 1979). This same report indicates that by the time American women reach age 60, upwards of one-half have had a hysterectomy. The net effect of the warnings, however, has been to limit the options of menopausal women who experience hot flashes or other menopausal body and/or affective changes by removing the one and only effective way of obtaining relief—through estrogen replacement.

Removal of estrogens from the menopausal woman's armamentarium of coping strategies has merely intensified the need to answer questions regarding the normalcy, homogeneity, or universality of the menopausal experience among women and the meaning of menopause associated changes.

MENOPAUSE AS NORMAL

If we depart from the medical literature, menopause is viewed from a different perspective. Margaret Mead saw menopause as an energetic, creative time in a woman's life. To her, the most creative force in the world was a menopausal woman with zest.

A changing perspective on menopause is also apparent in a growing body of literature, written by feminist researchers, which discusses menopause objectively and positively and raises important questions regarding the propagation of myths and fallacies about menopause, the preponderance of research against women, and makes explicit a need for interdisciplinary collaborative research using a woman-centered perspective in order to understand and redefine menopause for women. For example, the majority of feminist scholars do not append their findings to existing literature, nor do they strive to adhere to existing conceptual or theoretical frameworks to guide or support research questions. Instead, feminist scholars set about to critique existing theories and to generate a new literature altogether in which women are not just another focus but the center of an investigation whose categories and terms are derived from the world of female experience. Using a woman-centered framework then, menopausal women are not seen or defined as floating in a man's world; rather they are viewed as a coherent group—a context within themselves (Jehlen, 1981).

An example of the need to develop a new literature is provided by Adrienne Rich (1976). Rich said:

> Women have been both mothers and daughters but have written very little on the subject. The vast majority of literary and visual images of motherhood come to us filtered through a collective or individual male consciousness.
> As soon as a woman knows that a child is growing in her body she falls under the power of theories, ideals, archetypes,

descriptions of her new existence, almost none of which have come from other women.

Jo Ann Ashley (1978), a nurse, provides another example:

> Women are beginning to realize that dead and dying theories about the nature of human behavior have failed to say much that is meaningful about the true nature of women. Theories and conceptual frameworks growing out of patriarchal thinking have been damaging to women's health, their self-image and their sense of well-being. But women are finally awakening and beginning to question theories in fields ranging from religion to economics to politics . . . women are no longer willing to go along with the limitations imposed on them by male-dominated traditions. Liberated women want to think freely, they want to develop their own theories to explain the realities of their world and to shape their ideals accordingly.

To date, however, there is little indication of either feminist or woman-centered impact on the universe of male discourse related to menopause. Until recently, menopause was not a popular topic of conversation. Generally, women, as they entered menopause, were seen as diseased, as hopeless, confused, despairing, depressed, and quite sexless people.

While the situation has changed somewhat regarding attitudes toward menopausal women and the routine use of estrogen replacement has been discarded as a way of staying feminine forever, clinical journals in their advertising continue to project an image of the typical menopausal woman as worried, with wrinkled forehead, looking sad, and despairing over ugly aging liver spots. Menopause is seen as a time of confusion and frustration, a time in which counseling can help but can't stop vasomotor or vaginal symptoms, or retard bone loss. In some journal ads menopausal women are not seen as sexless. They are portrayed, however, as being unable to be sexual beings unless they are on estrogen replacement since it is inferred that a normal sexual relationship is not possible because of dyspareunia due to a cracked and bleeding vagina, without estrogen replacement.

And this image does not only exist in drug ads, it appears in professional journals too. When woman's child-bearing service has ended, her future, and indeed her destiny without estrogen replacement has been likened to spending the remainder of her life in a sort of living decay. It was this kind of grim picture that was painted by Robert Wilson in the 1960s, writing in a geriatric journal he said:

> The unpalatable truth must be faced that all postmenopausal women are castrates . . . . From the practical point of view a man remains a man until the end. The situation with a woman is very different, her ovaries become inadequate early in life . . . . A large percentage of women who escape severe depression or melancholia acquire a vapid cow-like feeling called a negative state. It is a strange endogenous misery . . . . Most of the suffering can now be prevented and effectively treated . . . . Because of custom and the lack of knowledge of these physical changes their presence and importance may be overlooked even in those close to us. Yet once the veil is lifted it is remarkable how quickly the previously uninitiated can detect these unfortunate women. Our streets abound with them—walking stiffly in twos and threes, seeing little and observing less. It is not unusual to see an erect man of 75 vigorously striding along on a golf course, but never a woman of this age. (Wilson & Wilson, 1963).

MacPherson (1981) in her excellent article, "Menopause as Disease: The Social Construction of a Metaphor," conceptualized the attitudes toward menopausal women in economic terms:

> From the pharmaceutical industry's viewpoint there was an enormous potential market for synthetic estrogen. The ovaries of all women eventually stop producing estrogen and synthetic forms of estrogen could be sold as a treatment to half the population for approximately 30 years of their life.

OUR MENOPAUSAL HERITAGE

The metaphor of menopause as disease has very deep roots. Let us share with you rather briefly our heritage. In 1850 we find written:

> Compelled to yield to the power of time, women now cease to exist as the species and henceforward live only for themselves.

Their features are stamped with the impress of age, and their genital organs are sealed with a signet of sterility. The first advice they ought to receive is to reject all sorts of drugs and receipts that are loudly proclaimed by ignorance and puffed by charlatanism. They ought not to sleep upon feather beds nor in any bed that is too soft and too warm, for such are attended with the disadvantage of exciting the generative organs which should hence forth, be left, as far as possible, in a state of inaction.

It is the dictate of prudence to avoid all such circumstances as might awaken any erotic thoughts in the mind, such as the spectacle of lascivious figures and the reading of passionate novels. (Ricci, 1947)

Negative attitudes toward menopausal women persisted into the 1970s and 1980s. In *The Management of the Menopause and Post-Menopausal Years* we find:

I have always drunk to the toast *vive la difference* and it seems logical that we should, if possible, *preserve la difference.* I think it is interesting that in the Oxford French Dictionary the verb *preserver* is illustrated by the phrase . . . "God preserve you from this misfortune," and now that He has given it to women to live so much longer, has he also provided the wherewithal to protect them from the misfortunes of the menopause, the physical changes of which range from loss of libido to the Dowager's Hump. . . . Would it not be better in the Autumn of their lives to give these women some prospect of an Indian Summer of happiness rather than a Winter of discontent? (Cope, 1976)

Similarly, Kistner (1979), a well known gynecologist, wrote:

The premenopausal decade (roughly age 40-50) may be a difficult obstacle for many women. During this time the symptoms revolve about a deterioration of feminine physical attributes frequently flavored by an intense distaste for aging— patients notice flabby skin, sagging breasts, increased skin pigmentation of the hands, chest or face, and flabby musculature . . . the basic concept of management includes psychotherapy designed to educate, reassure and support the patient together with relief of distressing symptoms and correction of estrogen deficiency.

A CHANGED PERSPECTIVE

There is hope, however. In terms of our heritage, menopause was not viewed totally as an unnatural, pathological process. For many women prior to the popularity of Wilson (1966) and his feminine forever/estrogen forever philosophy, menopause was viewed by some as a natural physiological event, one that seldom required medical intervention.

Of more significance for contemporary women is a growing body of literature written by researchers who discuss menopause objectively, positively, and raise important questions regarding (1) the propagation of myths and fallacies of bodily reductionism; (2) the preponderance of research against women; (3) the need for interdisciplinary collaborative research using a woman-centered perspective in order to understand, redefine and reconceptualize the menopause as a normal developmental period for women (Voda, Dinnerstein & O'Donnell, 1982).

Contemporary researchers question the menopause as disease concept because of the belief that such an assessment has arisen from the biased and mistaken assumptions of clinicians who see a nonrepresentative sample of menopausal women in their offices, and about whom they later write books. In reality, when a random sample of women was asked their opinion of menopause, very few thought negatively of the menopause although some said it could be unpleasant (Neugarten, et al., 1963).

Throughout the menopause literature there is a discrepancy between what the physician observes and how women actually experience an event. Apparently it is not easy for the physician and the woman to communicate about menopause. In a recent Canadian study, 44% of participating women between ages 40 and 60 had never raised the question with their physicians, while 83% reported that they rely on books and magazine articles for information (Kaufert, 1980). Female investigators of the menopause, on the other hand, tend to be bombarded with questions from women about the menopause and the transitional period. Thus, it is not for lack of questions that the topic is not commonly raised in the doctor's office. The medical approach to explaining menopause appears to be inadequate for the majority of women, not only because in its present form it does not invite discussions, but because of the continuing emphasis by the medical establishment on menopause as a deficiency disease, one that needs to be treated. The wide variety of questions asked by women indicate that they want to understand what is happening to their bodies, they want information that allows them to be prepared, to be able to predict, and then to adapt to change.

The experimental approach to studying menopause using a random sample of women gathered for one or two occasions of blood sampling or measurement does not yield information about how long term changes and experiences, which is what the menopause transition is, nor is there an interest in the normal case, that is, women who experience an uneventful menopausal transition. It is by and large the normalcy that remains undocumented. Nevertheless, some inroads have been made.

WHAT IS MENOPAUSE?

Menopause is the normal closure to menstrual and reproductive life. More technically, the menopause is that point in time when women have had their last menstrual period (LMP). However, women are not officially menopausal until one year has passed since the LMP. If any spotting or menstrual show occurs during this one year period, counting must begin all over again. Further, any excessive or unusual menstrual flow or spotting after one year's time without a period should be checked out immediately with a physician or nurse practitioner. If a woman has her ovaries removed along with her uterus, she immediately becomes menopausal, no matter what her age. In this case there is a rapid transition into artificial menopause due to a precipitous, rather than gradual, drop in sex hormones.

Since the menopause is but a point in time, this definition is not useful to women except as it marks the end of vaginal bleeding. We know that body changes, such as the hot flash, can occur four to eight years prior to the LMP. The onset of body changes prior to the LMP marks entry into a period defined as the perimenopausal transition, a period which may range from 10-15 years. For women who do not experience body changes prior to the LMP, the onset of irregular menstrual cycles with variations in menstrual interval and the quantity and quality of menstrual flow indicate that the menopausal transition has begun (Treolar, 1981).

WHAT IS THE ROLE OF THE SEX HORMONES?

Estrogen and progesterone are sex steroids synthesized in women's bodies by the ovaries and released into the circulation. During the reproductive years (menarche through menopause) estrogen is produced by the ovaries and rises and falls cyclically. The concentration in the blood varies with the phases of the menstrual cycle. Prior to ovulation, estrogen is necessary to start the process of building up the uterine lining to receive a fertilized egg(s). Then, a peak of estrogen (17 β estradiol) is necessary about day 13 so that ovulation itself can occur. After ovulation, the concentration of estrogen falls rapidly but then starts to go up again. This postovulatory increase in estrogen is necessary so that both estrogen and progesterone can further prepare the uterus to grow and become a hospitable place for a fertilized egg to implant. If fertilization does not occur, on about day 23 or 24, both estrogen (E) and progesterone (P) levels fall. Without the direction of P and E the uterine lining no longer continues to grow. Instead, around day 26-28, it begins to shed the lining of cells it grew. Menstruation is the process of shedding the uterine lining. For women who do not get pregnant, menstruation is a normal monthly, periodic, predictable, and, usually, welcome event. However, even as menstruation occurs, the level of sex hormone estrogen has started to increase and the entire process begins all over.

Much of the women's lives are spent in a body that has become quite used to estrogen periodically rising and falling. For women experiencing a natural menopause, the time span of estrogen domination in the body is about 30-35 years.

WHAT HAPPENS TO WOMEN'S BODIES
AROUND MENOPAUSE?

The appearance of some bodily and affective changes are predictable and normal. Some changes appear well in advance of the LMP and persist for years after the LMP. As mentioned, it is now preferable to refer to the menopause as a transitional period, one that may span 10-15 years, rather than defining it as a single point in time, since women's bodies go through many biological and biochemical adjustments prior to and after the LMP. For some unknown reason, at about age 40 (although the process can begin earlier) the ovaries can no longer respond to stimulation by brain hormones to produce estrogen and progesterone. The result is that at times periods become irregular, with both short and long intervals (Trebar, Boynton, Bohm & Brown, 1967). When menstruation occurs during this period of irregularity there is a high probability that periods are anovulatory, that is, menstruation occurs without ovulation.

As women get closer to the LMP, during some cycles the levels of brain hormones will increase in the presence of the sex hormones. The significance of these hormone changes is that it is perfectly normal for women prior to the LMP to feel the effects of these changing and fluctuating hormone concentrations in the form of affective and/or bodily changes. For example, hot flashes and or night sweats may occur during regular menstrual periods. This is perfectly normal! It is not known for sure whether decreased estrogen at this time is responsible for the hot flashes and/or other menopausal changes, but it is known that as estrogen levels begin to fall and brain hormones increase women begin to experience changes in their bodies.

WHAT ARE THE MAJOR CHANGES?

Hot Flash

Approximately 89% of women who experience menopause naturally (have not had their uterus, ovaries, and tubes removed) experience some kind of hot flash (Feldman, Voda & Gronseth, Note 1). The cause of the hot flash is unknown but the phenomenon is being studied from a variety of perspectives and recently has been linked to pulsatile lutenizing hormone secretion. Briefly, the hot flash is a sudden perception of heat located within and/or on the body; the heat has an origin and a spread and may or may not be accompanied by a sweat or a color change (Voda, 1981). (The hot flash is described in detail in a pamphlet titled *Coping With the Hot Flash*, Voda, 1981.)

Vaginal and Urinary Problems

Some women report vaginal dryness (a primary function of estrogen is to lubricate the vagina) and thus painful intercourse. Burning and painful urination has also been reported. Also the phenomenon of stress or urge incontinence is not uncommon in women. Stress incontinence is the inability to retain urine on coughing, sneezing, running, jogging, while women with urge incontinence leak small quantities of urine prior to the active act of urinating. Voda (1981a) found that 75% of menopausal women experienced either stress or urge incontinence which was unrelated to childbirth or bladder pathology.

Bone or Joint Pain

Osteoporosis is bone-thinning or demineralization of the bone and is associated with menopause. Women who have a family history of osteoporosis and who are of small bony stature are at high risk of developing it. Osteoporosis makes bones prone to fracture and sometimes produces painful joints. The cause of bone thinning is unknown and the same process also occurs in men, but at a later age. The prevalence of osteoporosis is unknown, but it is higher in fair skinned, small boned, thin Caucasian women.

Depression and Nervous Symptoms

Some women do experience shifts in their emotions around menopause. These changes are usually not severe. Feminist research on this topic seems to suggest that menopausal depression and mood swings are not totally due to hormone fluctuations. Rather, mood changes are the result of all the physical (for example, sleep loss due to hot flashes), family, and personal changes occurring during the transitional period (Voda, 1982). During the menopausal years women are faced with the reality of growing older in a culture that values youth. Very often their children have left or will soon be leaving home. Responsibility for aging parents increases. Thus perimenopausal women are experiencing external as well as internal changes that may adversely affect mood.

SHOULD WOMEN USE ESTROGEN?

The decision to use estrogen, that is, estrogen replacement therapy (ERT), is complex and personal. The pros and cons are examined below.

Pro: Coping with Changes

Hot flashes. Estrogen does alleviate hot flashes. It is the only agent that completely eliminates them (Voda, 1981a). For those women who experience disabling hot flashes high doses of estrogen may be needed (more than 1.25 mgm/day) to obtain relief. High doses of estrogens taken over long periods of time (more than five years) increase the risks associated with estrogen use. Research indicates that when estrogen is stopped, the hot flashes return. Estrogen merely postpones passage through the transitional period.

Vaginal and urinary problems. ERT either by mouth or vaginal suppositories or creams can alleviate genitourinary changes. If women take ERT in a vaginal suppository or cream and use it daily, the estrogen is rapidly absorbed into the circulation and the effect is similar to that of taking it in pill form and carries with it the same risks. Some women use vaginal estrogen suppositories thinking that the effect remains localized. It does not. There are a variety of nonestrogen creams and jellies on the market that are quite effective for vaginal dryness. Some women use cocoa butter, unsaturated oils, and the like. These methods are described by Reitz (1977) in her book, *Menopause, a Positive Approach.*

Bone loss or osteoporosis. Estrogen use during menopause appears to arrest bone loss but never replaces lost bone, and even this benefit appears to be limited to three to four years (Marx, 1980). There are ways other than ERT for warding off debilitating osteoporosis. These include a diet that includes 1200-1500 mgm calcium per day (the amount of calcium contained in about a quart and a third of milk), regular exercise, and avoidance of cigarette smoking and heavy drinking. There is no way other than by radiographic methods (x-ray of bones in arms, spine, and joints) to diagnose early osteoporosis. The first indication of the presence of osteoporosis often is when a fracture occurs.

Con:

Estrogen use carries with it the risk of developing uterine and breast cancer, blood clots, liver tumors, and many other well documented side effects. Estrogen use post menopausally essentially stimulates uterine cells that have been preprogrammed genetically to shut down. By taking estrogen, women are stimulating aged cells. The consequences of overstimulation of aged cells may result in a transformed cell which is the precursor of neoplastic or precancerous cell-types. To take estrogen cyclically as if to mimic a menstrual period is ludicrous since first—women are no longer cycling and do not have the same hormonal milieu, and second—withdrawal of estrogens for one week does not result in vaginal bleeding.

Other Concerns of Women

Other concerns of menopausal women surround the relationship between menopause and pregnancy, premenstrual tension (PMT), and premenstrual syndrome (PMS), dysmenorrhea, and menstrual periods in general. For example, women want to know if menopause will be earlier, longer, or more difficult if one experiences PMT, PMS, dysmenorrhea, multiple pregnancies vs. no pregnancies, or irregular menstrual periods?

It is known that some women suffer discomfort, tension, and irritability during the days immediately before menstruation. Many women also have a feeling of bloatedness and gain weight during this time. With the onset of menstruation the discomfort is relieved. A serious problem in studying menstrual phenomena is that the scientific status of the signs and symptoms that are said to comprise a premenstrual syndrome is very uncertain. As Parlee (1973) demonstrated a decade ago, it is extremely difficult to find any consistency in the definition of what constitutes PMS. It varies from woman to woman and frequently from period to period in the same woman. Furthermore, it has been extremely difficult to adequately document the changes that have been proposed to constitute the syndrome. This lack of definition partially explains the paucity of empirical data concerning whether there is a relationship between premenstrual changes and the menopausal experience.

The confusion surrounding PMS and PMT is in part due to the fact that some writers have drawn upon their clinical experience as the main source of information and, as a result, are more generous with definitive statements about possible correlations between premenstrual changes and the menopausal transition. Dalton (1978), for example, writes about women she has encountered. She assures her readers that sufferers of premenstrual syndrome (which in her view is a progesterone deficiency problem) will not suffer at menopause and thus will never need to consider estrogen treatment. Dalton also differentiates dysmenorrhea from PMS: dysmenorrhea is caused by too much progesterone in relation to estrogen, and dysmenorrhea sufferers will continue to suffer and in contrast to PMS sufferers will need estrogen to get through the menopausal miseries. Kistner (1973), a specialist in the field of managing menopausal women and a proponent of postmenopausal treatment, does not agree with Dalton's view of managing menopause for PMS women. He writes, ''A symphony of symptoms frequently occurs in the premenopausal female which are included in the 'premenstrual tension' syndrome of the younger female.'' Kistner ascribes the premenopausal woman's premenstrual problems to estrogen not progesterone deficiency. Cohen (1978), asserts that the signs of bloating, nervousness, and intestinal problems increase in frequency from adolescence on and become an almost constant presence during the years of premenopause. Three clinicians writing from three different national perspectives, Great Britain, the United States, and France, respectively agree on one thing—that there is a relationship between premenstrual problems and menopausal transition. There is no agreement, however, as to which direction this relationship takes.

Few empirical studies are available. One of the first large surveys of a normal sample of women in the menopausal years was done in Great Britain by the Medical Women's Federation (1933). Here a positive correlation was found between previous dysmenorrhea and menopausal problems of greater intensity.

Van Keep and Jazmann (1973) investigated a community sample of over 300 Swiss women who were post-menopausal (no menstrual periods for at least 12 months). More than 50% of these women reported menstrual-cycle related problems previously, and most had suffered from dysmenorrhea. However, there was no significant relationship between the presence of current menopausal problems and previous dysmenorrhea or premenstrual problems. More empirical data are needed before any answers to this important question of a relationship between previous menstrual-cycle related complaints and the menopausal experience can be offered.

Another question, one that appears simpler to deal with, concerns the relationship between reproductive history and menopause. Regarding age of menopause, there seems to be no conclusive evidence for a simple relationship between number of pregnancies and an early or late menopause. Thompson and colleagues (1973) could not find any such association in a sample of Scottish women and neither could Goodman and her co-workers (1978) who compared four ethnic groups in Hawaii. On the other hand, a study of menopausal age in women listed by general practicioners in London demonstrated a later menopause in women with several pregnancies (MacKinley & Thompson, 1972). However, this was true only in women of higher socioeconomic status, who had a later menopause than other women of similar parity. Also Ernster and Petrakis (1981) reported a later menopause in high-income women and in nulliparous (no previous pregnancies) women, as compared to poor women and to multiparous (more than one pregnancy) women. These writers speculated that the better nutrition in the women with high incomes contributed to a later menopause. Later menopause in women of high socioeconomic groups per se has also been reported by Jaszmann (Jaszmann, Van Lilth, & Zatt, 1969). However, very large and diversified samples of women need to be investigated to clarify this relationship.

The influence of earlier pregnancies on the quality of the menopausal experience is also of concern. In a large study of several thousand Dutch women age 40-60 it was found that women who had never been pregnant had fewer menopausal complaints (Jaszman, 1973). Sherman and colleagues (1981) studied women participating in a health screening project and divided them into two groups, women with and without hot flashes. All of the women were in menopause. In this comparison there were no differences between these two groups in either number of pregnancies, number of live births, or age at which menopause was attained. Here again studies of larger groups of women are needed in order to properly explore these complex associations.

Women also ask whether the age of menopause is related to age at menarche. Although biological processes are susceptible to environmental influence and the onset of menarche is now being reported as occurring at a younger age than years ago, probably because of improved nutritional conditions, menopausal age appears to be more firmly fixed. Studies of old records have determined that the average age for menopause has not changed appreciably since antiquity (Amundsen & Diers, 1970). Menopausal age has also been found to be remarkably invariant in different Western cultures, such as the Netherlands (Jaszmann, Van Lilth, & Zatt, 1969), Great Britain (MacKinley, Jeffrys, & Thompson, 1972), the United States (Treloar, 1981), and Sweden (Bengston, Lindquist, & Redwall, 1981).

In fact, it is claimed to be completely uninfluenced by culture. (Flint, 1975).

Given this background, we would expect no general relationship to be found between the age of menarche and menopause. And this seems to be the conclusion reached by most empirical investigators. Most studies, however, are naturally retrospective and, as such, may be frought with errors of recall, rounding off, etc. Nevertheless, no relationship has been reported between menarcheal and menopausal ages for a British sample (MacKinley, Jeffrys, & Thompson, 1972), a Dutch sample (Haspels & Van Keep, 1979), four different ethnic groups of women in Hawaii (Goodman, Grove, & Gilbert, 1978), and several American samples (Ernster & Patrakis, 1981; Sherman et al., 1981; Treloar, 1981). Treloar (1981), who conducted a rare prospective study of a large group of women from menarche to menopause, thus avoiding the problems of recall, also reports no association between age of menarche and age of menopause.

Other factors that alter the internal chemical milieu of women's bodies may influence the age of menopause. Smoking, for example, is reported to be associated with an earlier menopause (Kaufman, 1980). But what about the use of the pill? In recent years large groups of healthy women have been taking estrogenic compounds to prevent ovulation and/or to regulate their menstrual periods. It is reasonable to expect that pill use will have an effect on the perimenopausal transition. However, Goodman and her co-workers (1978) studying women of different ethnicity found no correlation between years of use of birth control pills and age of menopause, nor were there any differences between the groups studied. Sherman and associates (1981) similarly reported no association between age of menopause and years of use of oral contraceptives in women with menopausal hot flashes. Data from the Netherlands, however, tentatively suggests a later age of menopause in women who have had estrogenic compounds for many years (Haspels & Van Keep, 1979) and Treloar (1981) also found that women who had used estrogens (oral contraceptives and estrogen replacement) in the five years prior to menopause experienced menopause one to two years later than women who had not used estrogens. More details as to when the estrogens had been used, what kind of estrogens had been used, and when the women had stopped taking them are needed to clarify this important issue. Because of the prospective nature of Treloar's study and because his sample is so large, his data are more reliable than others. Thus, for the present, it appears that estrogen use of any kind delays the menopause. Unfortunately, other types of influence on the perimenopause due to estrogen use are unknown, for example is the severity and duration of the transitional period affected? This question has not been addressed.

Finally, large numbers of women will never experience the most common indication of the menopausal transition, that is a change in quantity and/or quality of menstrual flow, because their uteri were removed at an early age. If both ovaries and uterus are removed the woman will immediately experience menopause. Of concern here is the woman who has had her uterus removed but who has retained her ovaries, and whether this woman's menopause will resemble the menopause of a woman who has her uterus intact. There are difficulties involved in making a comparison of this kind since it is not possible to determine whether a woman is in the menopausal transition without the observable change in the menstrual periods. That is, for women who have had their uterus removed, it is no longer possible to use the last menstrual period as the criterion for becoming menopausal. Women who have undergone hysterectomy must then rely on body and affective changes to tell them that they have either entered or are in the transitional period. One of the most dramatic and prevalent body changes for these women is the onset of the hot flash.

Most writers are inclined to agree with Van Keep and Haspels (1979), who state, "If the ovaries have not been removed they will stop functioning at the age when natural menopause would have taken place anyhow." However, empirical investigations to substantiate this statement are rare. A recent study indicates that the age at which hysterectomy is performed is important. This study suggests that the older a woman is at the time of surgery, the higher the probability that she will enter early menopause after hysterectomy (Kaiser, Geiger & Kunzig, 1978). As indicated, more investigations of menopause are required in order to provide women with what they need to know about the changes to expect following hysterectomy.

A HEALTH PERSPECTIVE: WELL-BEING

Menopause is an objective event that can be recorded and assessed. It is also a subjective experience, creating observable physical alterations in women's bodies and it has the potential for affecting both their mental and physical health. There is growing concern that some menopausal women experience both a deterioration of physical health and depressive reactions to menopause (Eliasson, Note 2).

What can women do to foster their own well-being during the perimenopausal transition? Many menopausal women are involved actively with special diets, vitamin and mineral supplements, and regular exercise programs. These activities appear to have a positive influence on well-being. However, as yet no research is available to determine the extent of this influence. This is particularly problematic with regard to osteoporosis, a focal concern of menopausal women, because estrogen replacement for osteoporosis remains a controversial issue. Important questions remained unanswered. If osteoporosis can be induced by immobilization (Gordon & Vaughan, 1980), can it be prevented by exercising? Will calcium or other supplements prevent bone loss? The answers to these questions await further research. (Pamphlets that address frequently asked questions about osteoporosis, estrogen use, and the hot flash are available. See Voda, Note 3).

DIRECTIONS FOR FUTURE RESEARCH

A natural history of menopause is needed, a gathering of facts about menopause as a natural transition. Researchers must start from the beginning with cross-cultural investigations, in order to assess the way in which societal characteristics influence the menopausal experience; researchers need to study groups of individuals rather than stereotypes in order to avoid repeating the biased observations of the past. More than anything else, it is clear that continuing research on the menopause needs to be performed from a woman's perspective, utilizing information from women who are undergoing the experience. These women are the expert informants, and menopause must be defined out of that context. The use of a woman-centered perspective will enable researchers to avoid further biased observations and erroneous interpretations of such observations and will establish an open forum for the future.

REFERENCE NOTES

    1. Feldman, B.F., Voda, A.M., & Gronseth, E.G. Prevalance of menopausal hot flash. Unpublished report, 1981.
    2. Eliasson, M. Unpublished report.

3. Voda, A.M. Three pamphlets: Boning up for the menopause; To be or not to be an estrogen user; Coping with the hot flash. Available from: Ann M. Voda, PhD, University of Utah College of Nursing, 25 South Medical Drive, Salt Lake City, Utah 84112.

REFERENCES

Amundsen, D.W., & Diers, C.J. The age of menopause in classical Greece and Rome. *Human Biology*, 1970, *42*, 79-84.

Ashley, J.A. *Of women born.* New York: Bantam, 1976.

Bengston, C. Lindquist, O., & Redwall, L. Menstrual status and menopausal age of middle-aged Swedish women. *Acta Obstetrica Gynecologica Scandinavica*, 1981, *60*, 44-66.

Cohen, J. La syndrome premenstruelle. *Le Fait Feminin,* ed. Sullerot. Paris, Libraire Artheme Fayard, 1978.

Cope, E. Physical changes associated with the post-menopausal years. In S. Campbell (Ed.) *The management of the menopausal and the post-menopausal years.* Baltimore: Williams & Wilkins Co., 1978.

Dalton, K. *Once a month.* Glasgow: Fontana Paperbacks, 1978.

Ernster, V.L., & Patrakis, N.L. Effect of hormonal events in earlier life and socioeconomic status on age at menopause. *American Journal of Obstetrics & Gynecology*, 1981, *140*, 471-472.

Flint, M. The menopause: Reward or punishment? *Psychosomatics*, 1975, *16*, 161-168.

Goodman, M.J., Grove, J.S., & Gilbert Jr., F. Age at menopause in relation to reproductive history in Japanese, Caucasian, Chinese and Hawaiian women living in Hawaii. *Journal of Gerontology*, 1978, *33*, 688-694.

Gordan, G.S., & Vaughan, C. Prevention and treatment of postmenopausal osteoporosis. In N. Pasetto, R. Paoletti, & J.L. Ambrus, J.L. (Eds.). *The menopause and postmenopause.* Lancaster: MTP Press, 1980.

Haspels, A.A., & Van Keep, P.A. Endocrinology and management of the menopause. In A.A. Haspels, & H. Musaph, (Eds.) *Pscyosomatics in perimenopause.* Lancaster: MTP Press, 1979.

Jaszman, L., Van Lilth, N.D., & Zatt, J.C.A. The age at menopause in the Netherlands. *International Journal of Fertility*, 1969, *14*, 106-112.

Jaszmann, L. Epidemiology of climacteric and post-climacteric complaints. *Frontiers in Hormone Research*, 1973, *2*, 22-34.

Jehlen, M. Archimedes and the paradox of feminist criticism. *Signs*, 1981, *6*, 575-601.

Kaiser, R., Geiger, W., & Kunzig, H.J. Hormonstatus bei frauen nach hysterectomie im vergleich zu kontrollen. *Archives of Gynecology*, 1978, *226*, 363-368.

Kaufert, P.A. The perimenopausal woman and her use of health services. *Maturitas*, 1980, *2*, 191-205.

Kaufman, D.W. Cigarette smoking and age at natural menopause. *American Journal of Public Health*, 1980, *70*, 420-422.

Kistner, R.W. The menopause. *Clinical Obstetrics and Gynecology*, 1973, *16*, 106-129.

Kistner, R.W. The menopause. In R.M. Caplan, & W.J. Sweeny (Eds.) *Advances in obstetrics and gynecology,* Baltimore: Williams & Wilkins Co., 1978.

MacKinley, S., Jeffrys, M., & Thompson, B. An investigation of the age at menopause. *Journal of Biosocial Science*, 1972, *4*, 161-173.

MacPherson, K.I. Menopause as disease: The social construction of a metaphor. *Advances in Nursing Science*, 1981, *3*, 95-113.

Marx, J.L. Osteoporosis: New legs for thinning bones. *Science*, 1980, *207*, 628-630.

Molnar, G.W. Body temperature during menopausal hot flashes. *Journal of Applied Physiology*, 1975, *38*, 499-503.

Medical Women's Federation. An investigation of the menopause in one thousand women. *Lancet*, 1933, *1*, 186-187.

National Institutes of Health. Estrogen use and post-menopausal women. Report of NIH Consensus Development Conference Summary. NIH, Washington, D.C., 1979.

Neugarten, B.L., Wood, V., Kraines, R.J., & Loomis, B. Women's attitudes toward menopause. *Vita Human,* 1963, *6,* 140-151.

Parlee, M.B. The premenstrual syndrome. *Psychological Bulletin,* 1973, *80,* 454-465.

Reitz, R. *Menopause: A positive approach.* New York: Penguin Books, 1977.

Ricci, J.V. *100 years of gynecology.* Philadelphia: Blakeston Co., 1947.

Rich, A. *Of women born.* New York: Bantam, 1976.

Sherman, B.M., Wallace, R.B., Bean, J.A., Chang, Y., & Schlabaugh, L. The relationship of menopausal hot flashes to medical and reproductive experience. *Journal of Gerontology,* 1981, *36,* 306-309.

Smith, D.C., Prentice, R., Thompson, D.J., & Herrman, W.L. Association of exogenous estrogen and endometrial carcinoma amoung users of conjugated estrogens. *New England Journal* of Medicine, 1975, *293,* 1167-1170.

Thompson, B., Hart, S.A., & Durno, D. Menopausal age and symptomatology in general practice. *Journal of Biosocial Science,* 1973, *5,* 71-82.

Treloar, A.E., Boynton, R.E., Bohm, G.G., & Brown, B.W. Variation of the human menstrual cycle through reproductive life. *International Journal of Fertility.* 1967, *12,* 77-126.

Treloar, A.E. Menstrual cyclicity and the pre-menopause. *Maturitas,* 1981, *3,* 249-264.

Van Keep, P.A., & Jaszmann, L. Dysmenorrhoe, pramenstruelles syndrom und klimakterische beschwerden. *Geburtshilfe und Frauenheilkunde,* 1973, *33,* 669-671.

Voda, A.M. Climacteric hot flash. *Maturitas,* 1981a, *3,* 73-90.

Voda, A.M. *Coping with the hot flash* (pamphlet). Minnesota: University of Minnesota, 1981b.

Voda, A.M., Dinnerstein, M., & O'Donnell, S. *Changing perspectives on menopause.* Austin: University of Texas Press, 1982.

Wilson, R.A., & Wilson, T.A. The fate of the nontreated postmenopausal woman: A plea for the maintenance of adequate estrogen from puberty to the grave. *Journal of the American Geriatric Society,* 1963, *11,* 347-362.

Wilson, R.A. *Feminine forever.* New York: M. Evans, 1966.

Ziel, H.K., & Finkle, W.D. Increased risk of endometrial carcinoma among users of conjugated estrogens. *New England Journal of Medicine,* 1975, *293,* 1167-1170.